FIRST PLACE BIBLE STUDY

A NEW CREATION

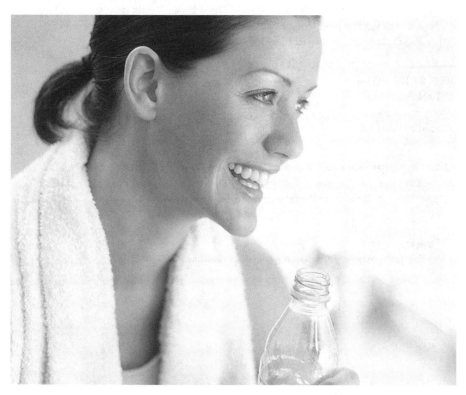

Gospel Light

FIRST PLACE™

Gospel Light

Gospel Light is a Christian publisher dedicated to serving the local church. We believe God's vision for Gospel Light is to provide church leaders with biblical, user-friendly materials that will help them evangelize, disciple and minister to children, youth and families.

It is our prayer that this Gospel Light resource will help you discover biblical truth for your own life and help you minister to others. May God richly bless you.

For a free catalog of resources from Gospel Light, please contact your Christian supplier or contact us at 1-800-4-GOSPEL or www.gospellight.com.

PUBLISHING STAFF

William T. Greig, Publisher • **Dr. Elmer L. Towns,** Senior Consulting Publisher • **Jessie Minassian,** Editor • **Bayard Taylor, M.Div.,** Senior Editor, Biblical and Theological Issues • **Rosanne Moreland,** Cover and Internal Designer • **Susan Sowell,** Contributing Writer

Songs: Written and produced by David Miner. Musicians: Joe Bergman, Chris Eddy, Gary Ishee, Sam Kallaos, Ken Lewis, Phil Madeira and David Miner. Vocals: Jonathan Allen, Chris Eddy, Alex Harvey, Phil Joel, Renee Martin, David Miner and Kate Miner. Voice-overs: Kate Miner and D. David Morin. Mastered by Joey Turner.

ISBN 0-8307-3356-6
© 2004 First Place
All rights reserved.
Printed in the U.S.A.

CAUTION
The information contained in this book is intended to be solely informational and educational. It is assumed that the First Place participant will consult a medical or health professional before beginning this or any other weight-loss or physical fitness program.

CONTENTS

FOREWORD

My introduction to Bible study came when I joined First Place in March of 1981. I had been in church since I was a small child, but the extent of my study of the Bible had been reading my Sunday School quarterly on Saturday night. On Sunday morning, I would listen to my Sunday School teacher as she taught God's Word to me. During the worship service, I would listen to our pastor as he taught God's Word to me. Digging out the truths of the Bible for myself had frankly never entered my mind.

Perhaps you are right where I was back in 1981. If so, you are in for a blessing you never dreamed possible. As you start studying the truths of the Bible for yourself, you will see God begin to open your understanding of His Word. Bible study is one of the Nine Commitments of the First Place program. The First Place Bible studies are designed to be done on a daily basis. Each day's study will take approximately 15 to 20 minutes to complete, but you will be discovering the deep truths of God's Word as you work through each week's study.

There are many in-depth Bible studies on the market. The First Place Bible studies are not designed for the purpose of in-depth study. They are designed to be used in conjunction with the other eight commitments of the program to bring balance into our lives. Our desire is for each member to begin having a personal quiet time with God each day. This time alone with God should include a time of prayer, Bible reading and Bible study. Having a quiet time is a daily discipline that will bring the rich rewards of balance, something we all need.

A part of each week's study is the Bible memory verse for the week. You will find a CD at the back of this Bible study that contains all 10 of the memory verses for the study set to music. The CD has an upbeat tempo suitable for use when exercising. The songs help you to memorize the verses easily and retain them for future reference. If you memorize Scripture as you study, God will use His Word to transform your life.

Almost every First Place member I have talked with about the program says, "The weight loss is wonderful, but the most important thing I have received from my association with First Place is learning to study God's Word."

God bless you as you begin this exciting journey toward a balanced life. God will richly bless your efforts to give Him first place in your life. Remember Matthew 6:33: "But seek first his kingdom and his righteousness, and all these things will be given to you as well."

Carole Lewis
First Place National Director

Introduction

The First Place Bible studies were developed to be used in conjunction with the First Place weight-loss program. However, the studies could also be used by anyone who desires to learn more about God's Word and His will, with the added bonus of learning more about living a healthy lifestyle.

A Balanced Life

First Place is a Christ-centered health program, emphasizing balance in the physical, mental, emotional and spiritual areas of life. The First Place program is meant to be a daily process. As we learn to keep Christ first in our lives, we will find that He is the One who satisfies our hunger and our every need.

God's Word contains guidelines for maintaining our physical well-being, equipping us mentally to make right choices, providing emotional stability to handle everyday circumstances as well as crisis situations and growing spiritually as we deepen our relationship with Him.

The Nine Commitments

The First Place program has Nine Commitments that will help you draw closer to the Lord and aid you in establishing a solid, consistent and healthy Christian life. Each commitment is a necessary and important part of the goal of First Place to help you become healthier and stronger in all areas of your life—living the abundant life He has planned for each of us. To help you achieve growth in all four areas, First Place asks you to keep these Nine Commitments:

1. Attendance
2. Encouragement
3. Prayer
4. Bible reading
5. Scripture memory verse
6. Bible study
7. Live-It plan
8. Commitment Record
9. Exercise

The Components

There are 6 distinct components to this Bible study to aid you in bringing balance to your life. These components include the 10-week Bible study, 4 Wellness Worksheets, 2 weeks of menu plans, the leader's discussion guide, 13 Commitment Records and the Scripture Memory Music CD.

The Bible Study

Each week of each 10-week Bible study is divided into five daily assignments with Days 6 and 7 set aside for reflections on the week's lesson. The following guidelines will help make your study more enjoyable and profitable:

- Set aside 15 to 20 minutes each day to complete the daily assignment. It's best not to attempt to complete a week's worth of Bible study in one day.
- Pray before each day's study and ask God to give you understanding and a teachable heart.
- Keep in mind that the ultimate goal of Bible study is not only for knowledge but also for application and a changed life.
- First Place suggests using the *New International Version* of the Bible to complete the studies.
- Don't feel anxious if you can't seem to find the *correct* answer. Many times the Word will speak differently to different people, depending upon where they are in their walk with God and the season of life they are experiencing.
- Be prepared to discuss with your fellow First Place members what you learned that week through your study.

Wellness Worksheets

This study's Wellness Worksheets are interactive and will help you further explore the topic of becoming a new creation in Christ.

Menu Plans

The two-week menu plans were developed especially for First Place by Chef Scott Wilson. Each menu is meant to simplify meal planning and include food exchanges. These meals are based on the MasterCook software that uses a database of over 6,000 food items and was prepared using United States Department of Agriculture (USDA) publications and information from food manufacturers.

Leader's Discussion Guide

This discussion guide is provided to help the First Place leader guide a group through this Bible study. It provides information for the leader to prepare for each weekly group meeting.

Personal Weight Record

The Personal Weight Record is for the member to use to keep a record of weight loss. After the weigh-in at each week's meeting, the member will record any loss or gain on the chart.

Commitment Records

Thirteen Commitment Records (CRs) are provided in the back of this Bible study. For your convenience these have been printed on perforated paper so that you can easily remove them from the book and carry them with you through each week as you keep your First Place commitments. Directions for filling out the CRs precede those pages.

Scripture Memory Music CD

Since Scripture memory music is such a vital part of the First Place program, the Scripture Memory Music CD for this study is included in the back inside cover. The verses for this study are set to music that can be listened to as you work, play or travel. The CD can be an effective tool as you exercise since the first verse is set to music with a warm-up tempo, the next eight verses are set to workout tempo, and the music of sthe last verse can be used for a cooldown.

WHAT IS A NEW CREATION IN CHRIST?

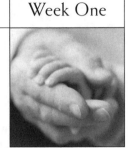

Week One

MEMORY VERSE

We were therefore buried with him through baptism into death in order that, just as Christ was raised from the dead through the glory of the Father, we too may live a new life.

Romans 6:4

The apostle John said, "I have no greater joy than to hear that my children are walking in the truth" (3 John 1:4). God also receives great joy in knowing that His children are standing on a foundation built by His truth—the Word of God. Every day that we base our thoughts, feelings and decisions on anything other than God's Word, we miss out on the tremendous blessings of living the way God created us to live. God gave us new lives when we accepted His priceless gift of salvation, and we are no longer slaves to our old ways of thinking, believing and living—we have been newly created!

DAY 1: *Above All Else*

If we truly desire to experience the life-changing power of God in our lives, then we must begin this study with an expectant heart. We must seek God, believing that He will be found. Hebrews 11:6 tells us, "Without faith it is impossible to please God, because anyone who comes to him must believe that he exists and that he rewards those who earnestly seek him." Notice the word "earnestly." God tells us to earnestly seek Him; to seek Him with intense desire.

➤ Have you ever sought after something with intense desire? If so, what did you seek? (You may list more than one thing.)

I feel like I do seek to please God
my children
Weight loss + health

What was your reward for seeking that thing?

I am still seeking, but I have joy & peace in doing that.
I wonder about that sometimes
I'm not there yet, but I've learned a lot.

As a member of First Place, you may have a strong desire to reach your weight-loss goal. If you follow the Nine Commitments of the First Place program, you will reach that goal and you will be rewarded in each step in the process. As we seek to live as new creations in Christ, we will be rewarded throughout the journey with His presence, His strength, His unconditional love, His grace and His joy.

Take a few moments to ask yourself, *Am I earnestly—with intense desire—seeking God?* Pray that today you will begin to seek God with an intense desire, knowing that He will reward you by revealing Himself to you.

Dear Father, I know that without faith it is impossible to please You [see Hebrews 11:6]. In faith, I desire to earnestly seek You. As I do so, I ask You to reveal Your truth to me.

DAY 2: *A New Foundation*

Yesterday we discussed the importance of seeking God. Before we begin today's lesson, please take a moment to ask God to draw near to you. Tell God that you want to know Him and that you desire His presence in your life.

Second Corinthians 5:17 says, "Therefore, if anyone is in Christ, he is a new creation; the old has gone, the new has come!" The moment you accept Christ as your Savior, pray and ask Jesus into your heart, you get a new life. At the moment you enter into relationship with Christ, your life becomes brand-new—your identity changes. You are no longer identified by the world's standards and views. You are not identified by your occupation, your position, your background, your mistakes or failures, the opinions of others or your opinion of yourself. Your identity is now given to you on the basis—the foundational truth—of your new relationship with Christ.

⋙ Read Acts 9:1-20. Describe in your own words what kind of experience Paul had with Christ.

v. 3
6

Paul was going to Damascus and gathering any Christians he could find along the way as prisoners. Christ appeared to him in a bright light. He spoke to him & changed his life

What do you think changed Paul's mind about the identity of Jesus?

meeting Christ and knowing the truth changed his life. He believed, got saved and was used of God (v. 15 - a chosen vessel)

Paul was presented with the truth. Paul came face-to-face with the One who *is* truth. Jesus said, "I am the way and the truth and the life. No one comes to the Father except through me" (John 14:6). Paul met truth face-to-face and yielded to the power that was revealed to Him through Jesus Christ, the Word of God made flesh (see John 1:1). That encounter caused Paul to change the way he regarded Christ, others and his own life. In the same way, when we encounter the Word of God, it will cause us to change how we regard Christ, others and ourselves.

⋙ According to 2 Corinthians 5:15-16, how did Paul's encounter with Christ affect the way he saw others?

He saw them thru (the way) Christ saw them

Do you tend to use a worldly point of view or God's Word to form your beliefs about God? About others? About yourself?

I always use The Word to form my beliefs about God? but not always about others & myself.

⋙ How do you think forming your beliefs based on the foundation of God's Word would affect your success in meeting your First Place goals?

It would be the difference between success & failure

Are you ready to form your beliefs about God, other people and yourself on the basis of God's Word? If so, ask God to help you begin to see yourself and your life through the truth of His Word. Write your prayer in the space below or in your journal.

Dear Father
I feel unworthy of your grace and mercy, but I know You can help me form my beliefs (are the only one who) about You, others and myself. Help me as I read + study Your Word to absorb your truths and apply them to my life and I need to start today.

DAY 3: *Our New Identity*

Yesterday we learned that we are to look to God's Word—not the world— to form our beliefs about Christ, others and ourselves. God's Word must be the source of and the authority over all our thoughts and beliefs. God gives us our identity and purpose in life.

➤ Read 2 Corinthians 5:17 again. What condition must be met in order to become a new creation?

If we have not committed our hearts and lives to Christ, then we are not in Christ and, therefore, cannot be newly created. Salvation is necessary before our identity can change.

If you have never given your life to Jesus Christ, you can pray and ask Him into your heart right now. You can have a brand-new life here on Earth and the promise of eternal life in heaven. All you need to do is ask. Tell Jesus that you need Him, and ask Him to be the Lord of your life. He loves you and will accept you just the way you are.

Yesterday you were asked, "Do you tend to use a worldly point of view or God's Word to form your beliefs about yourself?" Let's do a quick inventory. In the following chart, list some of the thoughts and beliefs about yourself and your life that you have on a regular basis. Next to each thought or belief, write whether the thought or belief originates from a worldly or biblical viewpoint.

some people have these thoughts

Thought/Belief	Origin
1. I'm not good enough	Worldly
2. I have to work hard to earn salvation	wordly
3. Jesus died for ME I'm valuable	Biblical
4. Jesus keeps me saved	Biblical
5. I can do all things thru Christ	Biblical

me

Read Ephesians 4:17-24. Paul is writing this letter to the church in Ephesus. In this part of the letter, Paul is giving the church instructions on how to live as God's children.

➤ In verses 17-19, of what does Paul warn us?

a hardened heart

In verse 18 we read, "They are darkened in their understanding and separated from the life of God because of the ignorance that is in them due to the hardening of their hearts." Our hearts can become hard as a result of experiencing pain and loss, or when sin resides within the walls of our hearts.

➤ Are there parts of your heart that have become hardened and as a result separate you from the knowledge of God's love for you? Explain. *No. You can't sit under Pastor's preaching or spend time in the Word and have a hardened heart*

Look again at verse 22. The word "corrupted" in Greek is *phtheiro*. It means "to destroy, perish; to be led astray."[1] We receive a new identity when we accept Christ as our Savior, but we still have an old self that needs to be put in its rightful place. The old self is no longer our identity, but if we let it retake control of our lives, it will destroy us. It will cause us to stray from the teachings of Christ and take us right back to our old ways of thinking, believing and living.

➤ How does your old self operate? What kind of desires does your old self have (v. 22)?

deceitful lusts

Our old self is not very smart, and it's no wonder—it does not have the knowledge and truth of Jesus. Our old self desires things that it thinks are necessary to make us feel better (e.g., food, praise, material things); but we are disappointed to discover that those desires were deceptive. The thing we have craved is not as fulfilling as we had thought and hoped it would be, and we ended up feeling defeated.

➤ What three instructions does Paul give us concerning our new self (vv. 22-24)?

Put off your old self
Be made new in the attitude of your mind
Put on the new self

Why is it important to follow these three instructions?

So as not to feel defeated
To be more like Christ
For the inner peace + joy that comes by obedience.

➤ In verse 24, how is your new identity described?

Created to be like God in true righteousness + holiness

Close today's lesson by asking God to remove any walls that have hardened your heart to the knowledge of His love for you.

Dear Father, I want more than anything to live as the new creation You desire me to be. Help me put to death my old self with its deceptive ways so that I can live in freedom. Thank You, God, for offering me this new life.

DAY 4: *A New Life*

Begin today's lesson by reading Romans 6:1-4. The word "grace" in verse 1 originates from the Greek word *charis*, which means "the state of kindness and favor toward someone, often with a focus on a benefit given to the object; gift."[2] God's grace is favor freely given to us for our benefit, and it is unconditional. God gives us grace based on who He is, not who we are. This unconditional grace is not what the world teaches about favor and kindness and giving. The world says that we have to perform well in order to receive favor, but God gives us grace because He loves us and because He is full of mercy.

⟫ In what ways do you struggle with receiving and applying God's grace in your life?

I sometimes struggle, as I think we all do w/sin. I am so thankful for 1 John 1:9 I never doubt my salvation, just accepting God's blessings on my life.

Most people have difficulty accepting God's grace. Our enemy, Satan, fills our minds with his lies to keep us from accepting this precious gift.

⟫ What thoughts do you have regarding God's favor, forgiveness, gifts and love that oppose the definition of God's grace?

Romans 6:3 states, "All of us who were baptized into Christ Jesus were baptized into his death." Baptism symbolizes that we have died to our old life and have been given a new one. Recall from our study of 2 Corinthians 5:17, "Therefore, if anyone is in Christ, he is a new creation; the old has gone, the new has come!" Baptism also symbolizes the death and resurrection of Jesus Christ. Jesus died and then rose from the dead three days later. Jesus conquered and has victory over death.

➤ According to this week's memory verse, Romans 6:4, what happened to your life at the moment of salvation?

We have new life

What is so significant about this verse in regards to your identity?

I am a new person. I have the power thru Jesus Christ to be anything He wants me to be

Jesus was raised from the dead through the glory of His Father. According to our memory verse, God uses the same power, His glory, to give us new lives. The Greek word for God's glory, *doxa*, has a wide range of meanings in the New Testament. It means "splendor," "brilliance" and "the awesome light that radiates from God's presence," and it is associated with His acts of power, honor and praise.[3]

➤ What does this truth tell you about your life the moment you received salvation?

I have new life

How was your old life put to death?

The new life took it's place

How were you given a new life?

By Jesus Christ

➤ How can you apply what you have learned today to the Nine Commitments of First Place and experience victory in the areas of health and fitness?

Phil 4:13 - I can do all things through Christ

Close today's lesson by reading Psalm 100 aloud as a prayer of praise to God.

Dear Father God, I praise You for conquering death through Your Son Jesus Christ. My old life has been put to death, and now I can live a new, victorious life because of Your marvelous grace. Teach me to rejoice in that knowledge.

DAY 5: A Crucified Life

Recall from this week's memory verse that at the moment of salvation, we figuratively die with Christ on the cross. Today we'll explore what it means to live a crucified life.

➣ Read Galatians 2:20-21. According to verse 20, what has happened to your life?

I no longer live, the old me was crucified

When did this happen?

The moment I accepted Christ

Now who lives in you?

Christ

A crucified life—that is what being a new creation in Christ is all about. Christ took our old self, put it to death on the Cross and gave us His life in exchange! Hallelujah! No wonder we can no longer consider ourselves from a worldly point of view.

➣ Reread Galatians 2:20. How can you embrace the powerful truth of your identity?

By faith in the Son

➣ How does Philippians 1:21 apply to your identity as a new creation in Christ?

We live not our own life, but the life Christ gives us.

➤ How does learning about your identity in Christ affect the way you see your success in First Place?

I can accompolish my goal, because I have the power of Christ in my new life.

Father, thank You that my old self is dead and that I have a new identity. You have given me new life and I am a new creation in Christ. Jesus, teach me to walk in Your truth. I want to bring You joy and bless You as I receive Your grace and power to free me from unhealthy thoughts and habits.

DAY 6: *Reflections*

This week we have been introduced to what it means to be a new creation. We are discovering through God's Word that each of us has an identity that isn't based on what the world teaches. Our identity—who we truly are—is not based on outward appearance, material possessions or our career. Our identity is based on who God says we are. When we begin to see ourselves the way that God sees us, we will experience great freedom from the damage that the world's teachings have had on our self-esteem.

We can be tempted to seek approval from other people and to be motivated to change in the hopes of receiving approval from them. The world certainly teaches us that being beautiful and thin will cause others to like us more. We are bombarded with messages that lead us to think that we need the approval of others and a perfect appearance in order to feel good about ourselves.

Are you motivated to eat healthily and exercise to gain approval from others? If so, allow Christ to help you begin to change by revealing your unhealthy thoughts, feelings and motivations.

If your motivation in joining First Place is to receive approval from others, confess that unhealthy motivation to Jesus. Ask Jesus to help you accept that your identity is in Christ and that God's perfect love and acceptance of you is what you need—not others' approval.

Father, thank You that Your way is perfect and Your Word is flawless [see Psalm 18:30]. I am in awe of You and desire to walk in Your ways [see Psalm 128:1]. Thank You that the Holy Spirit is guiding me to walk in Your truth [see John 16:13].

I invite You to search my heart and thoughts to see if there is any offensive way in me [see Psalm 139:23-24]. Lead me away from thoughts and feelings that offend You, and lead my heart and mind to seek and follow hard after truth.

DAY 7: *Reflections*

Just like Bible study, prayer is essential in growing closer to God. Prayer is simply speaking to God and listening for His answers. Prayer builds an intimacy with God that cannot be attained through any other means. Prayer is life changing, not only because it moves the hand of God, but also because it reveals the heart of God. It is no accident that we get too busy and too distracted to spend intimate moments in prayer with God. Satan knows how powerful prayer is, and he does everything he can to keep us off our knees.

In Old Testament times, people erected altars in honor of the one they worshiped. Altars were used to offer sacrifices, were places of prayer and served as reminders of God's promises. Abram built an altar to God in Genesis 12:7. Abram had just spoken with God and was compelled to build something in remembrance of his communion with God. Building an altar—a place of remembrance—provided a special place for him to visit when he wanted to remember the words God had spoken to him.

Ask God to show you a place to build an altar, a special place where the two of you can meet to share your hearts; a place where you can be still and remember the things that God has done for you; a place where you can worship God through your words or silence. Abram made his altar with rough stones and earth. You can use anything to make your place special or use nothing at all. Your altar could be in a closet, in the yard or at some other place in your home. Your altar's location and appearance are insignificant. Having a special place to be alone with God will help you develop a greater intimacy with Him.

Father, thank You that whoever dwells in the shelter of the Most High will rest in the shadow of the Almighty [see Psalm 91:1]. You are "my refuge and my fortress, my God, in whom I trust" [Psalm 91:2].

Father, Your faithfulness is my shield, my rampart and my defense [see Psalm 91:4]. Thank you that You will answer me when I call on you, that You will be with me in times of trouble and that You promise to deliver and honor me [see Psalm 91:15].

Notes
1. James Strong, *The Strongest Strong's Exhaustive Concordance of the Bible* (Grand Rapids, MI: Zondervan Publishing House, 2001), Greek #5351.
2. Ibid., Greek #5485.
3. Ibid., Greek #1391.

NAME	REQUEST	RESULTS
Jamice	Ann Boyer friend adam stomach cancer	
Leah	Parents visiting	
Carol	Betty Deskins brain surgery tomorrow	
Tamara	Lesley McElroy	
	Jim Dean	

DESIRE TO LIVE AS A NEW CREATION

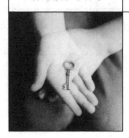

MEMORY VERSE
*Delight yourself in the LORD and he will
give you the desires of your heart.*
Psalm 37:4

The word "desire," as used in Psalm 37:4, means, "to express a wish for."[1] "Petition" is an action word that means, "to make a request."[2] When we desire to live as new creations in Christ, we are asking God for something that He very much wants us to receive. God wants to reveal Himself to us. God wants us know His Son. God wants us to know His great love, His abundant mercy and His plan for our lives.

DAY 1: *Battling Sin*

We learned last week that a new creation in Christ is a life that has been newly created by God at the time of salvation for the purpose of living in the image of Christ. We learned that the way we live in the image of Christ is to allow Him to live through us, and in order for Christ to live through us, we must choose daily to walk in the new identity we have been given.

Read Romans 7:14-25. This passage illustrates the battle that goes on between our sinful nature and our newly created identity. Can you relate to what Paul is saying? Have you ever not wanted to do something, but as much as you didn't want to do it, you did it anyway? As members of First Place, we want to follow the Nine Commitments, but that's not something we can do without God's help.

❧ Take a few moments to list the areas in your life in which you have this internal struggle—the battle between what you know you should do and what you actually do.

Prayer + Bible reading.
Judging others - compassion

❧ Look closely at verse 15. Are there physical or spiritual things that you really want to do but just do not seem to have the time or a strong enough commitment to do? Explain.

I want to see others as Christ sees them. I want to react to them always the way Christ would. In moments of stress I seem to be harsh, instead of loving + kind.

❧ Based on verses 18-20, describe our sinful nature.

not a good thing!

Notice that in verse 19, Paul states that he wants to do good and not do evil, but he continues doing evil in spite of his desire to do good. We may have a strong desire to eat healthily and exercise regularly, but our desire alone will not give us the strength we need to make our desire a reality.

❧ Read verses 21-24. Paul was describing an ongoing battle between his desire to do good and his sinful nature. Where was this battle taking place?

Inside himself

How did Paul feel during this battle?

He felt like a wretched man.

Our sinful nature is strong! Our godly desires alone will not conquer sin in our lives. We may desire to make the right food choices, but that by itself won't get us very far for very long.

➤ According to verse 25, who rescues us?

God through Christ

➤ Read Revelation 19:11-16. How is your mighty hero pictured?

As King of Kings + Lord of Lords

Take a few moments to write a prayer to God in the space provided or in your journal. Tell Him that you need Him and that you want His power to be revealed in your life to enable you to choose right over wrong. Be honest about any specific areas in which you need help in order to be successful in reaching your First Place goals. Surrender each and every desire to Him.

Dear Father,
You know that I am unworthy of your love and mercy, but I plead the blood of Jesus Christ. I am so thankful for You in my life. Without you I would be nothing. I need Your power to keep me pure and useable. Control every part of me, so that others will see You at work and glorify You. Help me to fulfill my First Place committments.

DAY 2: *Putting Christ First*

God wants to be the most important person to us, and He wants our relationship with Him to be the most important part of our lives. This requires sacrifice. We must desire intimacy with Christ in order to be willing to make those sacrifices. God knows what we need to sacrifice. He knows what we have allowed to take precedence over Him, and that we struggle to desire Him above everything and everyone else. God knows what we have become too dependent on in our lives.

➤ Read Luke 18:18-30. What was this rich young man seeking (v. 18)?

Eternal life

➤ How did Jesus respond to the man?

Sell everything and follow me.

Why do you think Jesus did not simply tell the man how to receive salvation?

He knew what was important to him.

Why do you think Jesus told the man to sell everything the man owned and to give it to the poor?

Riches were important to him. More important than Jesus.

➤ Jesus promised the rich young man treasures in heaven, or eternal life—the very thing the man had come to Jesus seeking. How did the man respond (v. 23)?

He was very sad

What was the man's stronger desire: treasure in heaven or material wealth?

material wealth

❧ Reread verses 24-25. Why do you think Jesus said these words to His disciples?

Jesus knows where our treasure is, what motivates and rules our life. The rich young ruler chose to trust in. riches

❧ How are stubborn barriers removed in our lives (vv. 26-27)?

By the power of God.

Have you given Christ first place in your life, or have you allowed self-made securities to become more important than He is? Ask God to examine your heart and show you the things that compete with Him for first place in your life.

We can't conclude the study of this passage of Scripture without seeing the reward of surrendering all and putting Christ first in our lives.

❧ In verses 29-30, what does Jesus promise us?

Many times more and eternal life.

Father, I want your Son to be the most important person in my life, though I confess that at times I seek other things in my life before Him. Teach me and guide me as I make the necessary changes to give Christ first place in my life. With You, Father, all things are possible. Thank You for giving me all the strength that I need.

DAY 3: *Kneeling in Prayer*

As we learn about our new identity and the importance of desiring to live as a new creation, our ultimate desire must be Christ Himself. We must desire to know Him and have Him consume our lives with His presence.

We learned on Day 1 that "desire" is an action word. One of the primary ways we can actively pursue Christ is through prayer—on our knees.

The Bible tells us of many godly individuals who were quick to bend their knees in prayer. Let's examine a few examples.

≫ Read Ephesians 3:14-19. What does Paul ask God to give his Ephesian brothers and sisters in Christ?

Power to grasp the love of CHRIST and to know this love that surpasses knowledge — that ye may be filled to the measure of all the fullness of God.

≫ Read James 5:17-18. For what extraordinary thing did Elijah pray?

that it would not rain (No rain 3½ years) that it would rain (it did)

≫ According to Daniel 6:10, how often did this man of faith devote time to prayer and worship?

3 times a day

≫ For a lesson in prayer from our greatest example, Jesus Christ, please read Luke 22:39-41. What can we learn about prayer from these verses?

Jesus had a usual (chosen) place of prayer He prayed alone He knelt down

≫ In what ways can you identify with these men and women of faith?

They all prayed They prayed for specific requests They prayed regularly

In what ways do they challenge you?

To pray for (His) power to understand the Word Pray for needs Pray often Have a special place

We see from Scripture that godly men and women actively pursue God on their knees. We even see our precious Savior seeking His Father on His knees. There are times when we are in need of God's help, we are in need of intercession for a loved one, we need strength to endure difficult circumstances, or we simply want to shut out the world around us and enter the quiet presence of our Lord. Other times we need to love Him and exalt Him as Lord over all.

➣ In Psalm 95:6-7, what does the psalmist beckon us to do?

Bow down in worship

To conclude today's lesson, go to the special place—the altar—you chose in week one and kneel before God in prayer. You don't have to pray in a certain position—just do what comes naturally. Spend as much time as you have praying to God. Tell God that you need Him and desire to know Him. Seek Him with all your heart.

 Father God, I am seeking You with all my heart. I ask You to give me Your Spirit of wisdom and revelation so that I may know You better. Open the eyes of my heart so that I may know the hope to which I am called, the riches of Your glorious inheritance and Your incomparably great power [see Ephesians 1:17-19].

DAY 4: *Preparing to Delight*

There are some things that need to happen in our hearts before a strong desire for Christ and a new life in Him can begin to develop. We learned yesterday that desiring to know God means that we actively pursue Him. Today we will study Scriptures that teach us how to prepare our hearts for our pursuit to know God.

➣ According to Psalm 37:4, our memory verse for this week, what must happen before the Lord will give us the desires of our hearts?

We must delight in Him

The Hebrew word for delight, *anog*, can mean both "to be delicate" and "to delight."[3] When we delight in the Lord, we are tender toward Him. Our hearts are soft toward God because He is so precious to us. In week one, we learned about the danger of having hard hearts.

In Ephesians 4:17-19, what does Paul warn believers to avoid?

a hardened heart

According to verse 18, what is the result of having a hard heart?

Our understanding is darkened, we withdraw from God (spiritual death)

Sin is not the only root of a hard heart. Pain and loss can also cause our hearts to become hardened. We may even blame God for our pain and loss and become angry with Him. It is during those times that we truly need the knowledge of God. We need to know that He understands and loves us and will heal and deliver us. Our ignorance of these truths results in a hard heart (see v. 18).

What are we promised in 1 John 1:9?

If we confess our sin, He is faithful and just to forgive us our sin.

How does this verse apply to a hard heart?

I think your heart has to be softened to confess your sin. A hardened heart will not see (realize) sin

Ask God to show you if there are areas in your heart that have become hard toward Him. Invite God to reveal any sin in your life and allow Him to show you any wounds that need His healing. Close today's lesson by spending time talking to—and *listening* to—God. You may want to spend this time at your altar.

Father God, keep my heart from becoming hardened by sin's deceitfulness. Protect my heart from turning away from You because of sin and unbelief. Help me to encourage others to hold firmly till the end with confidence [see Hebrews 3:12-14].

DAY 5: *Cultivating a Tender Heart*

Yesterday we learned that our hearts need to be prepared for the desires that God wants to place within us. Having a tender heart toward God is absolutely essential as we begin to live as new creations.

↬ In the space provided, write Psalm 37:4 from memory.

"Delight thyself also in the Lord; and He shall give thee the desires of thine heart."

In biblical language, the heart governs the intellectual, *(mind)* emotive, *(emotions)* voli-tional and physical dimensions of the inner person.[4]
(will)

↬ How are our hearts described in Proverbs 4:23?

The wellspring of life

What are we told to do with our hearts?

Guard them

Why do you think we are given this instruction?

If the heart ~~tells~~ rules all these, we should certainly guard it.

↬ From what specifically do you need to guard your heart?

from hardening before the Lord.

How can you guard your heart from those things? Be specific.

listen to God (read His Word)
talk to God (pray)
meditate on Him

Phil 4:9

Act. 13:22 – a man after God's own h.

I Sam 16:7 the Lord looketh on the h.

Prov. 4:23 Keep thy h. w/all diligence out of it are issues of life

mt. 12:34 Abundance of h. the mouth speak.

Mt 15:19

- God desires us to study His Word (see Psalm 1:2). *His delight is in the Law of the LORD*
- God desires to comfort and heal us (see Psalm 34:18) *The Lord is nigh unto them of a broken heart.*
- God desires us to receive salvation (see John 3:16). *For God so loved*
- God desires us to worship Him in spirit and in truth (see John 4:23). *But the hour cometh, when true worshippers shall worship the Father in spirit and in TRUTH; for the Father seeketh*
- God desires to bless us with a fulfilling life (see John 10:10). *... I am come that ye might have life more abundantly*
- God desires us to walk in freedom (see Galatians 5:1). *Stand fast in the liberty where Christ hath made us free.*
- God desires us to be filled with the fruit of the Holy Spirit: love, joy, peace, patience, kindness, goodness, faithfulness, gentleness and self-control (see Galatians 5:22-23).

- God desires that we find joy in Him, pray and give thanks at all times (see 1 Thessalonians 5:16-18). *Rejoice evermore. Pray w/o ceasing. Give thanks in everything= God's will*
- God desires us to confess our sins and receive forgiveness (see 1 John 1:9). *If we confess our sins, He is faithful + just to forgive us our sins*
- God desires us to walk in the truth of His Word (see 3 John 1:4). *I have no greater joy than to hear my children walk in truth.*

These are just some of the many desires that God has revealed to us in His Word. Satan will certainly lie to us and tell us that desiring the things close to God's heart will not be fun, rewarding or satisfying. The truth is that Satan came to steal our joy, our peace and our freedom. But God sent Jesus to give us abundant life. Our God is full of blessings and has poured them out to us through the gift of His Son. We have been given new life—we are new creations!

Dear Father, thank You for revealing Your desires for me in Your Word. I rejoice in the blessings You have showered on me! Continue to teach me what it means to live as a new creation in Christ.

Notes

1. *Merriam-Webster's Collegiate Dictionary*, 11th ed., s.v. "desire."
2. Ibid., s.v. "petition."
3. James Strong, *The Strongest Strong's Exhaustive Concordance of the Bible* (Grand Rapids, MI: Zondervan Publishing House, 2001), Hebrew #6026.
4. *International Standard Bible Encyclopedia*, vol. 2 (Grand Rapids, MI: William B. Eerdmans Publishing, 1982), s.v. "heart."

GROUP PRAYER REQUESTS   TODAY'S DATE:_____

NAME	REQUEST	RESULTS

CHOOSE TO LIVE AS A NEW CREATION

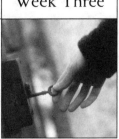

MEMORY VERSE

Since, then, you have been raised with Christ,
set your hearts on things above, where Christ is
seated at the right hand of God. Set your minds
on things above, not on earthly things.

Colossians 3:1-2

As we have learned, we are given new lives in Christ at the time of salvation. Because Jesus died on the cross at Calvary, we are forgiven of our sins and now have freedom from our past life. God gives us our new identities by His grace; however, we must choose daily to what or whom we will bow down and serve. We will either succumb to our old thoughts, beliefs and way of life, or we will choose to live as new creations in Christ.

DAY 1: *A Yielded Heart*

God used Joshua to lead His people, the children of Israel, into the Promised Land. God had delivered the Israelites from slavery in Egypt, but before long the Israelites turned their backs on God once again. After spending 40 years wandering in the desert, the Israelites were finally allowed to enter the land God had promised them.

Read Joshua 24:1-27, keeping in mind that Joshua was speaking to people who belonged to God. Joshua urged the people to renew their love and commitment to God and reminded them of the many things that God had done for them.

➤ List some of the things that God did for His Chosen People.

He led Abraham out of a land that worshipped idols
He brought them out of Egypt

V.13 *He parted the Red Sea to rescue them*
He gave them victory after victory to Caanan
He gave them a land for which they did not labour, cities they did not build, vineyards & oliveyards they did not plant

➤ What did Joshua command the people to do (vv. 14-15)?

Fear the Lord, serve Him in sincerity &
in truth; put away idols.
Choose you this day whom ye will serve.

➤ How did the people respond to Joshua's commands (vv. 16-18)?

The Lord is our God, therefore we
will serve the Lord.

➤ Why do you think Joshua rebuked their response (v. 19)?

Maybe he thought they were not sincere,
he wanted them to realize that
God would know.

➤ After the people chose to serve God, what two things did Joshua instruct them to do (v. 23)?

Get rid of your idols, and give
your heart to God

What do you think it means to yield our hearts to the Lord?

Our heart means our inner being,
everything we do and feel and say
reflects our heart. God wants all that.

Joshua 24:15 is a popular verse. However, we don't hear the verse preceding it very often.

➤ Write verse 14 in the space provided.

Now therefore fear the Lord, and serve
Him in sincerity and in truth. And
put away "idols" and serve the Lord.

➤ What two specific instructions are we given in verses 14-15? Why do you think we are given the instructions in this order?

Psm
19:9

I think if we don't have this "fear" we
won't want to serve Him

fear = reverential trust w/hatred of evil

↠ Read verse 15 again and notice what Joshua told the people about their desires. What does our desire have to do with our decision to serve God?

Choose you this day whom you will serve. There must be a desire before there will be service

We learned last week that God will place His desires in our hearts, but we must first delight in Him. Sometimes we have to choose to be obedient and serve God before we will feel the desire to please Him.

↠ How do you think choosing obedience until you receive the desire to be obedient can help you reach your First Place goals?

Obedience leads to desire to reach our goals

Lord, "Your word is a lamp to my feet and a light for my path" [Psalm 119:105]. It stands firm in the heavens for all eternity [see Psalm 119:89].

Father, I choose to delight myself in You while I wait patiently for You to place Your desires in my heart. I choose to serve You this day, and I choose to walk in the truth of Your unfailing Word.

DAY 2: *A Clean Heart*

God must come before anyone, or anything else, in our lives. Yesterday we learned through our study of Joshua 24 that we make a daily choice whether to yield our hearts to God. When we choose to yield to and serve God, we are choosing to live as new creations in Christ. Today we will continue our study of Joshua 24, focusing on a second command that God gives us.

↠ For review, list the two commands Joshua gave the people of Israel in Joshua 24:23.

Get rid of your idols, and give your heart to God.

Turn to Exodus 32:1-6 and read an account of the Israelites' unfaithfulness to God and their rejection of Him, even after He delivered them from slavery.

≫ When did the Israelites choose to make an idol?

It is easier to serve an idol, than to serve God, is is less demanding. God wants our whole being.

? ≫ Why do you think they made a foreign god to worship?

Any idol would be a foreign God? Maybe they thought a foreign God wouldn't know much about them.

The following is a list of things that can become idols in our lives. These are comforts we turn to instead of turning to God, masters we serve instead of serving God, idols that can become more important in our lives than God. Notice that most of the items on the list are blessings from God and need to be a part of our lives, but they are not intended to take the place that is reserved for God—first place.

- Achievement
- Alcohol and drugs
- Anger
- Exercise
- Fear
- Food
- Hobbies
- Money
- Relationships
- Shopping
- Sleep
- Television
- Volunteer work
- Work
- Worry

Do you have a tendency to put any of the idols on the list in God's rightful place? As we close today's lesson, spend some time in prayer. Ask God to examine your heart and life and to show you what needs to be removed and what needs to be devalued. In the space provided or in your journal, write down what God reveals to you about your life.

Lord,
I want to be all Yours. Show me if anyone or anything else comes before you in my Life. I love You, I want to serve you in spirit & in truth. I need Your wisdom & power to do that.

Precious Father, I want You to sit on the throne of my heart where You belong. Show me the things that compete with You for first place in my life. I want to have an undivided heart for You.

DAY 3: *An Extended Heart*

Through our study of Joshua 24, we have learned that we must choose to serve God daily and to tear down the idols that keep us from God. Today let's look at what it means to extend our hearts to God.

➤ For review, read Joshua 24:14-23. What two things are we instructed to do in verse 23?

Get rid of idols and serve God.

The *King James Version* says to "incline your heart" to God. The Hebrew word for incline, *natah*, can mean "to spread out, stretch out; be extended."[1] To incline our heart to God means that we are extending it out to Him.

➤ Can you imagine stretching and reaching your heart out to God? What thoughts and feelings come to your mind?

You may really struggle with the thought of reaching your heart out to God. You may question whether God will accept your heart, or perhaps you fear that He will not grab hold of you. Many things can affect how we view God's love for us.

➣ Do you question or doubt God's love for you? Explain.

Never

➣ Read 1 John 3:1. Based on this verse, describe God's love for you.

Great love

Song "The Love of God"

➣ According to 1 John 4:9, how did God demonstrate His love for us?

He sent Jesus, His only Son to die for me.

➣ Read Romans 8:38-39. What do these verses tell us about God's love for us?

Nothing can separate us from His love

To close today's lesson, please write a prayer to Jesus in the space provided or in your journal. Extend your heart to Him—pour out your feelings. Allow this to be an intimate time between you and your precious friend and Savior.

Dear Father,
You know my heart better than anyone. Search me and know my thoughts. Show me how to be strong for you. Reveal to me what I am really like and forgive me. Thank you for loving me so much in spite of my unfaithfulness to Your Person.

DAY 4: *An Undivided Heart*

We have been learning that choosing to live as new creations in Christ means choosing to give Christ our hearts and lives, choosing to give God first place in our lives. Just as Joshua challenged the Israelites to offer God more than lip service, God also challenges us to make a sincere and strong commitment to Him.

Recall from a previous lesson the biblical meaning of a heart. Our hearts are the center of the human spirit from which spring emotions, thought, motivations, courage and action. "Undivided" means "not separated into parts or pieces," or "united."[2]

⟫ Read Psalm 86:11. Using the biblical meaning of "heart" and the definition of "undivided," describe the kind of heart the psalmist is asking God to give him.

undivided heart - whole being - all parts wanting the same, yearning toward God!

⟫ In Ezekiel 11:18-20, what did God promise to give His children?

An undivided heart

What did God tell Ezekiel would happen before He fulfilled that promise?

They would remove all idols

⟫ What similarities do you see in Ezekiel 11:18-20 and God's instructions in Joshua 24?

*v. 14 Get rid of the idols
Choose to serve w/ undivided heart*

Figure 1 provides an example of both a divided and an undivided heart. Please use Figure 2 to list what creates a divided heart in you.[3]

Figure 1

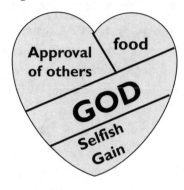

Divided Heart

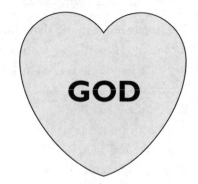

Undivided Heart

Figure 2

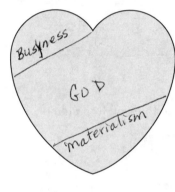

Divided Heart

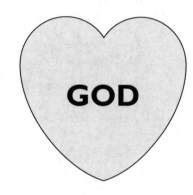

Undivided Heart

≫ Read Psalm 139:23-24. In your own words, explain what the psalmist asked God to do.

Search for divisions in his heart, heal them or show him how to.

≫ Look back at Psalm 86:11. Besides asking God to give him an undivided heart, what else did the psalmist ask God to do for him?

Teach me your way

What do you think is significant about the order in which the requests were made?

Teach + obedience = undivided
(knowing) (truth)   heart
WORD

Do you have a teachable heart? Are you willing to change the way you think and feel, what you do and what motivations you have? Are you willing to allow God to teach you His ways? If not, ask God to give you a teachable heart.

How did Jesus describe Himself in John 14:6?

I am the Way, the Truth, and
the Light

If we have teachable hearts, being confronted with truth will help us to change. If we have extended our hearts to God, His truth will set us free from our old thoughts, feelings and motivations, and our actions will begin to change.

Read John 8:31 and write Jesus' promise in the space provided.

If you obey my Word, you are
really my disciples.

Father, I thank You for sending Your Son, Jesus, to free me. Teach me Your ways and give me an undivided heart so that I can serve You and love You wholeheartedly.

DAY 5: A Heart of Worship

The meanings of the Hebrew word for serve, *abad*, include "to work, serve, labor, do; to worship."[4] When we choose to serve God whole-heartedly, we are also choosing to worship Him. The Hebrew word for worship, *saba*, means "to bow down."[5]

➤ What do you think it means to bow down in worship before God?

Our whole being recognizes the wisdom & knowledge of Him who made us!

How might worship be a form of serving God?

Without this wisdom & knowledge we can do nothing

➤ Read John 4:23. How does God want us to worship Him?

In Spirit and in truth

What do you think it means to worship in spirit?

Our whole being reaching out through the strength & power of His Spirit connecting

What do you think it means to worship in truth?

Know the truth and the truth shall set you free according to the Word. (Re: Uzzi)

God wants us to give Him our hearts and to serve Him wholeheartedly. He wants us to remove the things in our hearts that come before Him so that He can have first place in our lives.

➤ How do you think a heart extended to God in total service reflects the type of worship that God is seeking?

God is seeking willing obedience. If we obey Him because we love Him, I think God is pleased.

➤ How do you think we get to the place where we can worship God in spirit and in truth?

Spending time getting to know Him

➤ Spend a few moments thinking of ways that you have worshiped God in the past, as well as new ways you can worship Him. List them in the space provided.

praise   singing
obedience   giving
listening   serving

Father, teach me to worship You in spirit and in truth. I want to be the kind of worshiper that You seek. I want to please You by worshiping You with my life.

Show me, God, how to live a life of worship—not just once a week, but every day. Remove what stands between us so that I can worship You freely and wholeheartedly.

DAY 6: *Reflections*

This week we have learned that God wants us to choose to serve Him. Another word for "choose" is "decide." Our memory verse for this week is a great example of the choice we face regarding what we will focus our thoughts and hearts on. Our memory verse instructs us to do something with our thoughts and our hearts. Notice that the word "desire" is not included in these instructions! We must *choose* to obey—or disobey— the instructions in these verses. If we want to please God and reap the tremendous benefits of obedience, we will choose to set our hearts and minds on things above; we will decide to fix our eyes on Jesus, His truth and His purpose for our lives.

God, thank You for giving me Your Word and for blessing those who delight in Your law and meditate on Your law both day and night [see Psalm 1:1-2].

Father, I choose to fix my thoughts and my heart on You. I turn away from selfish desires and worldly gain. Thank You that Your truth sets me free.

DAY 7: *Reflections*

There is no faster way to put God in first place in our lives than to exalt Him through worship. I am convinced that God loves worship because of the deep intimacy it brings between Him and His beloved children. Worship ushers us into the throne room where God resides in all His glory. Worship touches the heart of God, which we could never do without His amazing grace, boundless love and endless glory.

Read the following words of the psalmist aloud in worship to your King of glory:

The earth is the LORD'S and everything in it, the world, and all who live in it; for he founded it upon the seas and established it upon the waters (Psalm 24:1-2).

For God is the King of all the earth; sing to him a psalm of praise. God reigns over the nations; God is seated on his holy throne (Psalm 47:7-8).

You are awesome, O God, in your sanctuary; the God of Israel gives power and strength to his people. Praise be to God! (Psalm 68:35).

How lovely is your dwelling place, O LORD Almighty! My soul yearns, even faints, for the courts of the LORD; my heart and my flesh cry out for the living God (Psalm 84:1-2).

O LORD God Almighty, who is like you? You are mighty, O LORD, and your faithfulness surrounds you (Psalm 89:8).

For great is your love, higher than the heavens; your faithfulness reaches to the skies. Be exalted, O God, above the heavens, and let your glory be over all the earth (Psalm 108:4-5).

Loving Father, thank You for allowing me to bless Your heart through worship. My heart is filled with longing for You, my King and my God. May the way I live my life reflect the love and devotion I have for You.

Other verses
David's psalm
I Chron.
16:8-9
v. 8-9
25
34
36

Notes

1. James Strong, *The Strongest Strong's Exhaustive Concordance of the Bible* (Grand Rapids, MI: Zondervan Publishing House, 2001), Hebrew #5186.
2. *Merriam-Webster's Collegiate Dictionary*, 11th ed., s.v. "un," "divided."
3. Beth Moore, *A Heart Like His* (Nashville, TN: LifeWay Press, 1996), p. 209.
4. Strong, *The Strongest Strong's Exhaustive Concordance of the Bible*, Hebrew #5647.
5. Ibid., Hebrew #7812.

GROUP PRAYER REQUESTS   TODAY'S DATE:_____

NAME	REQUEST	RESULTS

RECOGNIZE YOUR OBSTACLES

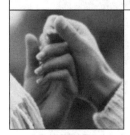

MEMORY VERSE

For I am the LORD, your God, who takes hold of your right hand and says to you, Do not fear; I will help you.

Isaiah 41:13

When we choose to serve God and begin to live as new creations in Christ, we are going to face some obstacles! This week we will look at several obstacles that we may face at one time or another. As we study these obstacles, remember that Jesus is already victorious over any obstacle we encounter, and because of the Cross, we have been given the power of Christ to overcome any obstacle that stands in the way of what has been given to us.

DAY 1: *The Obstacle Behind You*

Today we will examine an obstacle that can easily affect us in our pursuit to live as new creations: our past.

➤ Read Proverbs 3:5-6. What does God instruct us to do?

Trust in the Lord w/all my heart. Don't trust my understanding, but trust Him

What does God promise He will do when we follow His instructions?

He will direct my paths.

What does this verse tell you about every obstacle you encounter?

He will lead me around or through it.

⇨ Write Psalm 18:2 in the space provided. *The Lord is my rock, and my fortress, and my deliverer; my God, my strength, in whom I will trust; my buckler, and the horn of my salvation, and my high tower.*

The Hebrew word for deliver, *palat*, means "to escape; to rescue, deliver; to bring to safety, carry away safely; cause to escape."[1] God is our deliverer; He faithfully rescues us and brings us to His safety when we seek His shelter.

Sometimes there is no way around the obstacles we face; however, whether we walk through the obstacle or God provides a way around it, the end result is the same. God will deliver us and we will be free from the obstacle that stood between us and where God wants us to be. Whatever way our sovereign God chooses to lead us, we can be confident that He is faithful and that He plans to prosper us and to give us a hope and a future (see Jeremiah 29:11).

Read over the following list of potential obstacles and see if any of them are present in your life:

- Complacency
- Fear
- Food
- Grief
- Jealousy
- Laziness
- Pride
- Rejection

- Selfishness
- Sin
- Tragedy
- Unbelief
- Unforgiveness
- Unhealthy Relationships
- Worry

➤ List other obstacles that come to your mind.

family
busyness - can't say "No"

Our past is one obstacle that is not included on the list, yet it often contributes to many other obstacles. Wounded hearts have a difficult time walking in truth and experiencing freedom.

➤ Are there wounds from your past that hinder you? If so, what are those wounds?

There were some, but God has helped me work thru them.

How might those obstacles affect your ability to live as a new creation in Christ?

They might occupy your mind, so that you can't focus on what God wants for you.

We will spend time in weeks eight and nine learning how to allow Jesus to heal our wounds. For now, be encouraged that Jesus will heal every place in your heart and life that needs His touch.

➤ Read Isaiah 61:1-3. What does God desire us to receive to replace any wounds we carry from our past?

(beautiful) beauty for ashes
oil of joy for mourning
garment of praise for the spirit of heaviness

Thinking about painful experiences from our past can create many different feelings. For those with fresh wounds, those feelings may be uncomfortable. For those who have already been healed by God from a painful wound, thinking about His healing touch may create feelings of joy and gratitude.

Write a brief letter to Jesus in the space provided or in your journal. Tell Him what feelings are in your heart. Remember to thank Him for being your deliverer.

DAY 2: *The Obstacle of Busyness*

Getting to know a person requires spending time with him or her. During His time on Earth, Jesus clearly communicated how important it is for us to spend time with Him. Jesus wants us to know Him and to know Him intimately. He wants to reveal Himself to us.

➤ Read Luke 10:38-42. What was Martha doing and what kind of mood was she in?

Serving — I think preparing a meal
Stressed

What was her sister Mary doing?

Listening to Jesus
@ His feet

➤ What did Martha want Jesus to do for her?

make mary help her

Why did Martha ask this of Jesus?

She would have liked to be where Mary was - she was jealous - but felt her duty to serve was more important.

≫ In the space provided, write Jesus' words to Martha.

Martha, MARTHA, you are worried & upset about many things, but only one thing is needed. Mary has chosen what is better, and it will not be taken away from her.

≫ How do you think a few moments at Jesus' feet would have changed Martha's attitude?

Yes

Turn to John 12:1-3 and read another story of Martha and Mary. Once again we find Mary at the feet of Jesus.

≫ Is the scene different this time? If so, what differences do you see?

Not much, Martha's not complaining Mary's worship is different - listening & serving

If we desire to live as new creations in Christ, we must sit at the feet of Jesus or we will quickly become distracted and worried about insignificant things. Jesus said that only one thing is needed: to sit at His feet (see Luke 10:39,42). As we spend time with Christ, we are equipped by His grace to care for the other matters that need our attention.

Jesus taught us by example how to receive the strength, power and grace we need to be Christlike.

≫ Read Mark 1:35. When and where did Jesus go to pray to His Father?

A solitary place

Dear Father, I desire to know You intimately, and I know the only way to do that is to spend time with You. Show me ways I need to change my daily routine in order to spend more time with You.

Lord Jesus, give me a passion for You so that, like Mary, I will be found sitting at Your feet, lavishing You with my praise.

DAY 3: *The Obstacle of Unbelief*

As we spend time studying God's Word, we are presented with absolute truth. Every time that we read God's Word, we either choose to believe or reject what God is telling us. It may be easy to believe God's Word while we are reading it, but are our thoughts based on that truth throughout the day?

Let's do a little self-examination. What kind of thoughts have gone through your mind today? Of those thoughts, which ones have you spent time entertaining? What kinds of thoughts have you had concerning the challenges you face today? What kinds of thoughts do you have when you consider the Nine Commitments and your goals for First Place? In the space provided, list as many thoughts as you can identify.

① First thought – get up w/o too much pain
② Pray for a good bathroom visit
③ " for Janet – in hospital – call her
④ Talk to Mom first thing, so she won't feel left out.
⑤ Check weather – Richard traveling
⑥ Do this lesson, pray, fill in fact sheet
⑦ Get ready for work – plan the day.

➤ According to Philippians 4:8, about what are we to think?

Things that are noble, right, pure, lovely and admirable.

➤ Read Colossians 3:1-3. On what are we to set our minds?

On things above, where Christ is.

The Greek word for "set," *phroneo*, means "to think, regard, hold an opinion; to set one's mind on; to have a certain attitude."[2] Let's look at a few Scriptures that warn us of the danger of not setting our minds on things above.

➤ According to Romans 8:5-8, what is the result of a mind that is set on what the sinful nature desires?

death, hostility to God
Cannot please God.

➤ Read 2 Corinthians 4:4. How does Satan (the god of this age) work in unbelievers' minds?

So they cannot see the light of the Gospel of the glory of Christ

➤ Satan has been trying to make God's children doubt God's Word from the beginning of creation. Read Genesis 3:1 and write Satan's words below.

Did God really say?

➤ Based on what you have learned in Scripture today, how could the negative thoughts you listed earlier affect your success in First Place?

The "I can't do it" mentality is from satan and will never get us anywhere near success.

➤ How would doubting God's Word affect your success at living as a new creation in Christ?

Without His Word, we have nothing to sustain us.

Father, thank You for taking hold of my right hand and helping me. I know that I don't have to overcome any obstacle in my own strength. Your Holy Spirit is working in me to give me victory. I choose to believe that Your Word is true and that it will transform my life.

DAY 4: *The Obstacle of Pride*

Today's obstacle keeps many people from ever accepting Christ as their Savior. It keeps people in bondage to Satan's lies and has destroyed countless relationships. It creates a wall that prevents believers from seeking God earnestly and passionately. This obstacle is pride.

➤ Read Luke 18:9-14. To whom was Jesus telling this parable (v. 9)?

To some who were confident of their own righteousness and look down one everybody else

➤ What differences did you notice between the Pharisee's and the tax collector's prayers?

One was proud about himself The other was humble + desired mercy.

➤ Why did the tax collector go home "justified before God" (v. 14)?

Everyone who efaults himself shall be humbled Everyone who humbles himself shall be exaulted

➤ What do you think the Pharisee was seeking?

approval of man

➤ According to Galatians 1:10, what can rob us of being a servant of God? *Seeking for the approval of men*

Do you struggle with a desire to please others? Do you struggle with feeling as though you need others' approval? If so, ask God to help you experience freedom from this type of bondage. You may want to memorize Galatians 1:10 and allow this truth to help transform this area of your life.

Pride can be very subtle and is a master of disguise. For example, when we attempt to do things in our own strength, we are really saying that we can do them without God. When we act independently of God, we tell Him that we don't need Him. Remember, living as new creations in Christ means Christ lives through us. We do nothing on our own!

➤ List the things in your life that you attempt to do—either successfully or unsuccessfully—without Christ's help.

I can't think of anything - lose weight maybe

Have you ever considered it prideful to leave God out of these things? Why or why not?

Yes, without Him I can do nothing

➤ Read Luke 15:11-32. What lessons can we learn about pride from this story?

Is it more prosperous to lay down your pride

➤ According to Psalm 25:9 and Psalm 149:4, what blessings do the humble receive?

guidance in what is right salvation

➤ According to 1 Peter 5:5-6, what does God do for the humble?

He gives grace

➤ Read James 4:10. What does God promise to do for those who humble themselves before Him?

He will lift you up.

➤ How do you think pride could affect your success in reaching your First Place goals?

Give God the glory

➤ How could pride affect your success at living as a new creation in Christ?

Only if we are too proud to take instructions from God and think we can do it on our own

Go to your special place and kneel before God. Confess any areas of your life in which you harbor pride. Surrender those areas to God and make a decision to rely on His help and strength.

Father, I know that I am completely dependent on You for even the air I breathe. Cleanse my heart from any root of pride so that I can humbly serve You.

DAY 5: *The Obstacle of Overindulgence*

Indulging in a little too much of a good thing is an obstacle everyone can relate to. God certainly desires to bless His children and wants us to enjoy the gifts He gives us. However, God knows that we need guidance in order to live in this world and still remain devoted to Him. It is too easy to put material things, food, hobbies, relationships and desires before Christ.

Read Matthew 6:19-21. Verse 19 says, "Do not store up for yourselves treasures on earth." The word "store" is derived from the Greek word *thesaurizo* and means "to store up, gather, reserve; heaped treasure together."[3] The word "treasure" is derived from the Greek word *thesaurus* and simply means "what has been stored up or gathered together; storeroom."[4] What we spend our time and energy accumulating is what will be found in the storeroom.

➤ Why do you think Jesus tells us not to gather things for a storeroom on Earth?

Our treasures should be in heaven. On earth these things can be stolen or decay.

➤ Jesus said, "Store up for yourselves treasure in heaven" (v. 20). How is this heavenly storeroom described?

Where moth & rust do not destroy & theives do not break in & steal.

➤ What are the differences between a storeroom on Earth and a storeroom in heaven?

*Earthly - temporary
Heavenly - eternal*

➤ When you think of worldly treasures, what things come to your mind?

houses, cars, jewelry

➤ When you think of heavenly treasures, what things come to your mind?

*those you've lead to Christ
good deed done in the name of Jesus*

➤ Read Matthew 6:25-34. What does Jesus tell us in verse 33?

Seek first the kingdom of God and His righteousness

➤ According to 1 John 2:15-17, what things are of the world?

Cravings of sinful man
lust of the eye
boasting of what he has & does

lust of flesh
lust of the eye
pride of life

What will happen to the things of the world?

They will pass away

➤ Write Matthew 6:21 in the space provided.

For where your treasure is, there your heart will be also.

Recall that a treasure is "what has been stored up" or a "storeroom." Jesus is saying that our heart resides in the storeroom, among all the things that we have labored to accumulate.

➤ Read Matthew 6:22-23. What do you think Jesus is talking about?

What you look upon & desire - good or bad

➤ Read Hebrews 12:2. What instructions are we given concerning our eyes?

Fix your eyes on Jesus

Thank You, Father, for blessing me in the heavenly realms with every spiritual blessing in Christ [see Ephesians 1:3]. You have poured out Your blessings on my life through Your beloved Son.

Lord, give me the strength not to take Your earthly blessings for granted. I don't ever want to allow Your gifts to take first place in my life. That place is reserved for You alone.

DAY 6: *Reflections*

This week's memory verse is a wonderful promise to hearts that may feel overwhelmed after studying obstacles for five days! "For I am the LORD, your God, who takes hold of your right hand and says to you, Do not fear; I will help you" (Isaiah 41:13). God wants us to know that no matter what obstacles we face in life, He is equipped to handle them. He is Lord over everything, and He has power over our past, our present and our future.

Our memory verse also says that He is "your God." God wants us to know that, though He is big and mighty, He gave Himself to us. He is our Abba Father, our daddy.

The third point this verse makes is that God reaches down and grabs hold of His children's hands. Like a protective mother with a small child in a busy parking lot, God is quick to reach out to His beloved children.

"Your God . . . says to you" means that God speaks to our hearts. When we take time to see God as Lord of all and as our tender and compassionate Father, we will hear the words He speaks to our hearts with the love and grace with which they were spoken. His words will become what our hearts long to hear; they will silence the storms raging within us; they will encourage the weak and bring healing to the most wounded of hearts.

 God, I want to know You better. Enlighten the eyes of my heart so that I may know the hope to which You have called me, the riches of Your glorious inheritance and Your incomparably great power for me [see Ephesians 1:17-19].

DAY 7: *Reflections*

Learning to live as new creations in Christ, submitting our lives fully to the Lord, reaching goals we have set in First Place and experiencing healing and freedom in our lives are some of the things that God desires for us. These are some amazing and wonderful works of the Lord! God knows each of us and has a purpose and a plan for what He is doing in our individual lives (see Jeremiah 29:11). Spend some time in prayer thanking God for the many ways He ministers to your life, including the following ways:

- Lord, thank You for Your unfailing love and for the wonderful deeds You do for me [see Psalm 107:21].

- Thank You for giving me eternal life because I believe in Your one and only Son [see John 3:16].

- Thank You for sending forth Your Word to heal me and rescue me from the grave [see Psalm 107:20].

- Thank You for keeping me in perfect peace. My mind is steadfast because I trust in You [see Isaiah 26:3].

- Thank You for being my shepherd and supplying all my needs [see Psalm 23:1].

- Thank You that Your power is at work within me and that it can do immeasurably more than I can ask or imagine [see Ephesians 3:20].

- Thank You, God, for being my rock, my fortress and my deliverer. You are my shield and the horn of my salvation—my stronghold. Thank You for saving me from my enemies. You are worthy of praise [see Psalm 18:2-3].

I love You, Lord, You are my strength [see Psalm 18:1]. Thank You for revealing glimpses of Yourself through Your Word and through Your creation. I long for the day when I will stand in Your presence and worship You face-to-face.

Notes

1. James Strong, *The Strongest Strong's Exhaustive Concordance of the Bible* (Grand Rapids, MI: Zondervan Publishing House, 2001), Hebrew #6403.
2. Ibid., Greek #5426.
3. Ibid., Greek #2343.
4. Ibid., Greek #2344.

GROUP PRAYER REQUESTS TODAY'S DATE:_____

NAME	REQUEST	RESULTS

EXERCISE YOUR GIVEN AUTHORITY

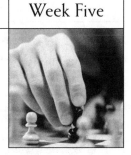

MEMORY VERSE
*For the LORD your God is the one who
goes with you to fight for you against
your enemies to give you victory.*
Deuteronomy 20:4

Last week we studied some of the obstacles that we face as new creations in Christ. This week we will study how to overcome those obstacles. Our enemy, Satan, does not want us overcoming obstacles. Satan attempts to rob us of abundant life by creating obstacles and then tempts us to doubt our ability to overcome them. He wants God's children to feel defeated. Jesus says that Satan "comes only to steal and kill and destroy; I have come that they may have life, and have it to the full" (John 10:10). Let's discover together the full life Jesus intends us to have.

DAY 1: *Connecting with Christ*

God has given us an incredible gift to overcome obstacles: God chooses to work in our lives and in the lives of others through our prayers.

➤ Read Luke 11:1-13. In verses 9-10, Jesus tells us to do three things in prayer. List those things and what He promises in return.

Ask - and it shall be given you
seek - and ye shall find
knock - and the door will be opened
to you

➤ What gift did Jesus say His Father will give those who ask (v. 13)?

Holy Spirit

What does this imply about other things for which you pray?

God will give us the good gifts

➤ In Jesus' parable, how does the man in need approach his friend? What is the result of his approach (v. 8)?

with boldness

➤ According to Hebrews 4:14-16, how are we to approach God (v. 16)?

with boldness-(confidence)

Why can we approach God in this way (vv. 14-15)?

Jesus, our high priest, is able to sympathize w/our weaknesses, having been tempted in every way we are.

Why do you think God wants us to approach Him in prayer in this manner?

Jesus died for me, He wants me to claim all the promises He gave when He suffered and died to fulfill them.

God gives us many promises concerning prayer. When we understand these promises, we are more likely to spend time in prayer. The more time we spend in prayer, the more we are connected to Christ. The more we are connected to Christ, the more we are living as new creations, so let's look at some of these promises together.

➤ Look up the following verses. Next to each verse, write the promise or benefit associated with prayer.

Results of prayer

Deuteronomy 4:7

God is near me when I pray to Him

Examples of prayer

2 Chronicles 7:14 - *If my people will humble themselves + pray, He will hear + forgive + heal*

Psalm 4:1 *Relief from my distress, mercy*

Psalm 86:6-7 *mercy / He will answer us*

We should pray

A New Creation

Proverbs 15:8 *The prayer of the upright pleases Him*

2 Corinthians 1:10-11
Deliverence, favor

Philippians 4:6 – *Don't worry about anything, tell God, but be thankful*
v. 7 = (promise) The peace of God will guard me
James 5:15-16 – *prayer offered in faith will make the sick, well.*
The prayer of a righteous man avails much

⇛ Based on these Scriptures, list some obstacles that can be removed through prayer.

Any obstacle you have can be removed through prayer.

⇛ How do you think spending more time in prayer would affect your success in First Place and as a new creation in Christ?

When God hears our prayers and obstacles are removed, then we have success.

Thank You, Father, for wanting to work in my life and to reveal Yourself to me through prayer. I want to spend time with You and seek Your provisions for my life through daily communication with You.

God, I ask You to create in me a hunger to spend time with You in prayer. Increase my understanding of prayer and teach me to pray as I should.

DAY 2: *Moving Mountains*

Some situations in our lives appear to be bumps in the road. Other situations seem to be huge mountains that we can't possibly climb. Regardless of the size of the obstacle in our lives, Jesus can move the mountain or give us the strength to climb it.

⇝ Read Matthew 17:14-20. What was the tremendous obstacle in the father's life?

Lack of faith

⇝ The man asked Jesus' disciples to heal his son. According to verse 20, why couldn't they heal the boy?

Lack of faith

⇝ Read Matthew 10:1. What authority did Jesus give those same disciples?

Authority to drive out devils and to heal every disease + sickness

The authority that Jesus gave His disciples was in His name (see Luke 10:17). Let's look at a few more verses that teach us how powerful that name is.

⇝ Read Philippians 2:9-10. What will happen one day at the very sound of Jesus' name?

every knee shall bow and every tongue shall confess that He is Lord

⇝ Read Acts 4:12. What is given to us through Jesus' name?

salvation

⇝ According to Matthew 18:20, what does Jesus promise?

Where two or three are gathered together, I am in the midst of them.

⇝ Look again at Matthew 17:20. What did Jesus tell the disciples they needed in order to move an obstacle (mountain)?

faith

At the time Jesus was speaking, the mustard seed was thought to have been the smallest seed. Under favorable conditions, this tiny seed could produce a plant 15 feet in height.[1] When we plant the seed of faith in our hearts and allow Christ to grow us, we can do the impossible—by the power that He has given us.

➤ In your own life, have you ever faced a mountain that Christ helped you overcome? Explain.

> Many mountains - still facing them Children's spirituality or lack of Personal mountains - God knows

➤ Are you facing a mountain in your life today? Explain.

Based on what you have learned today, how are you to respond to that obstacle?

> I am praying

In closing today, recall a mountain that Jesus moved in your life. In the space provided or in your journal, thank Him and praise Him for His faithfulness. Make a decision to trust Him to move any obstacle you are facing in your life today.

> Many years ago I faced a decision in my marriage that would affect my whole life. God carried me through that and has NEVER let me down.
> I wanted children. I agonized w/ God over this. He answed my prayed in His way).

DAY 3: *Kneeling at the Cross*

We are equipped with prayer, the name of Jesus and God's Word to overcome obstacles in our lives. Today we will allow God to examine our hearts
and reveal any obstacles that hinder us from living as new creations in
Christ. Spend a few moments in prayer to prepare your heart before you
begin today's lesson.

➤ Ask God to show you thoughts, feelings, behaviors, relationships or
any other obstacle that might be hindering you. List them in the
space provided.

thoughts - sometimes I rebell
feelings - I'm not all that bad
relationships - my youngest daughter

What are your thoughts and feelings toward those obstacles?

I am not happy.

Are your thoughts and feelings about those obstacles based on the
truth of God's Word? If so, list those thoughts and feeling below.

No -

➤ What do you think is the difference between knowing God's Word
and applying it to your life?

If you know you are sick, and have
medicine to take, but don't take it.
It's like knowing God's Word, but not

How do you think applying God's Word to your life would affect the
obstacles you face?

He promises to give me victory

We may find it difficult to allow God's Word to rule over our thoughts and feelings. Sometimes our own thoughts and feelings are the obstacles that we have the most difficulty overcoming. One of the ways we can allow God's Word to rule our thoughts and our hearts is through the love of Christ. The biggest obstacle we have ever faced was our spiritual separation from God. Because of the powerful love of Christ, we have overcome that obstacle through His death on an old, rugged cross.

➤ When you consider the death Jesus died for you, what thoughts and feelings do you have concerning the obstacles in your life?

> *He faced every obstacle and overcame them, so can I.*

➤ According to Romans 8:38-39, is there any obstacle that can separate us from God's love?

> *Nothing*

Do you ever struggle to accept that God's love for you is unchanging? If so, write Romans 8:38-39 on an index card and memorize that Scripture.

➤ For review, list the five obstacles we discussed last week that can affect our relationship with Christ.

> *past*   *pride*
> *busyness*   *overindulgence*
> *unbelief*

How do you think Christ's love can help you overcome each obstacle?

➤ Write down any specific obstacles that are keeping you from reaching your First Place goals.

How do you think Christ's love can help you overcome those obstacles?

If your heart is burdened, or if there is something creating a wall between you and Jesus, visit the Cross. Take a "Cross-trip." Close your eyes and extend your heart to Christ. Acknowledge His great sacrifice for you and accept the love that He yearns to give you. Then surrender your burden to Him. Leave it with Him at the foot of the Cross. Do not leave the Cross until you have completely given Jesus your burden. Then thank your closest friend and praise His holy name.

Father God, I give You praise and glory. Thank You for carrying my burdens each day of my life [see Psalm 68:19]. I am choosing to trust that You know my needs and that all my needs are met through Christ [see Philippians 4:19].

DAY 4: *Living by the Spirit*

Today we will study the fourth resource God had given us to exercise our given authority.

Read Ephesians 3:14-21. The apostle Paul was praying for his fellow Christians, and because this prayer is God's Word, we know that Paul was praying for what God desired them—and us—to receive.

➤ What does Paul ask God to give us (v. 16)?

power

Through whom does Paul say God will give us this gift?

Holy Spirit

We could spend weeks studying the Holy Spirit. For a quick overview of the work of the Holy Spirit in our lives, read John 16:7-15.

➤ According to these verses, what are some of the works of the Holy Spirit?

Convict the world of sin
guide you into all truth
He will tell you what is yet to come
He will bring glory to Jesus.

➤ According to Ephesians 1:13, when do we receive the Holy Spirit?

the same time we received Christ

➤ Read Romans 8:26-27. What is another way the Holy Spirit helps us?

He helps us pray - to know what to pray for.

➤ Read 1 Corinthians 2:11-12. What does this verse say about the Holy Spirit's role?

He reveals the things of God to us.

➤ Based on the Scriptures you have read today, describe the Holy Spirit.

He is a convictor   teacher
guide
intercessor

Read Galatians 5:22-23. The fruit of the Spirit is produced in a believer's life when the Holy Spirit is in control. *love, joy, peace, patience, kindness, goodness, faithful gentle self-control*

➤ Which fruit of the Holy Spirit do you especially struggle with attaining in your life? List any that apply.

self-control

➤ What do you think Paul meant when he said, "Live by the Spirit, and you will not gratify the desires of the sinful nature" (Galatians 5:16)?

read v. 17 For the sinful nature desires what is contrary to the Spirit & vise versa. They are in conflict w/ each other.

What things can you do daily in order to live by the Spirit rather than by the sinful nature?

pray, read the Word, sing, have others pray for me.

➤ What things might you be doing to hinder the power of the Holy Spirit in your life?

don't do any of these, get too busy

➤ What role does living by the Spirit play in successfully changing your eating habits?

He reminds me, when I am willing to listen

God, I am so grateful that because I belong to Christ Jesus, my sinful nature has been crucified with its passions and desires [see Galatians 5:24].

Lord, You are able to do immeasurably more than all I ask or imagine, according to the power that is at work within me [see Ephesians 3:20]. I give You praise and glory and honor.

DAY 5: Speaking Truth

God has fully equipped us to overcome any obstacles in our lives through His gifts of the Holy Spirit, prayer, His Word and His boundless love. We are indeed blessed! Today we will examine an integral part of our lives, our speech, and discover how our own words impact our lives as well as the lives of others.

➤ Read James 3:3-12. How does God describe the work of the tongue in these verses?

Small member, great power

➤ Where does the fire of the tongue originate (v. 6)?

Sin

➤ Read Proverbs 18:21 and 26:28. How do you think the enemy of our souls, Satan, works to destroy our lives through our own speech?

Death + life - a lying tongue = affliction I have a sharp tongue. I have to watch carefully and pray a lot to stay out of hot water.

➤ According to Ephesians 4:29, what kind of influence should our words have on others?

Your words should build up, encourage others.

➤ Read Ephesians 4:15. What is the benefit of speaking truth?

Maturity in Christ

➤ Based on these Scriptures, how do the words we speak affect our lives?

More than we want to think about.

Becoming aware of the power our words have over our lives is the first step in choosing to change our speech. The second step is recognizing speech that is harmful to us and to others.

➤ What things do you commonly say about your life that are not based on the truth of God's Word?

The third step in changing our speech is to replace the lies that we speak with God's truth. Look at the list of negative, or defeating, words you speak about your life. Next to each statement, write a Scripture that will encourage and strengthen you. Use more paper if necessary.

The final step in having victory over our speech is simply to begin speaking truth. We must make the choice to speak words that are based on God's Word and are 100 percent true, rather than words that are full of discouragement and doubt. Praise God that Jesus defeated Satan and that we have been given victory through Christ to speak life!

 Father, may every word that comes out of my mouth and every meditation within my heart be pleasing in Your sight [see Psalm 19:14].

God, You are my redeemer, and I ask You to deliver me from the deceitful power of my own tongue. Teach me to speak only what is beneficial to myself and to others.

DAY 6: *Reflections*

As we learned from our memory verse last week, God makes it clear who He is and that you belong to Him. The God of the universe chooses to be your personal Lord. The Hebrew word for Lord is *Yehwih* (pronounced YAH-way). Knowledge and use of the name Yehwih imply a personal or covenant relationship. Yehwih depicts God as the One who exists and causes existence.[2] When God tells us that He is our "Lord," it is a declaration of His covenant relationship with us; and a covenant relationship cannot be broken.

Now let's look at this week's memory verse. The Lord says that He is the One who goes with us to fight for us against our enemies (see Deuteronomy 20:4). That means we have someone on our side who knows all the strategies and plans of our enemy. God knows how to win the battle! Our commander is all powerful, and no weapon can stand against Him. He is also all present. God is with us every second of every day. God doesn't leave us for a moment to check on another set of troops. He is with each of His soldiers, right there fighting with them. We are guaranteed victory!

Take a moment to surrender any battle that you are facing to these truths about our God. Allow the truth of your memory verse to change the way you see your battles. Make a decision to say your memory verse out loud or silently any time the enemy tempts you to think untrue thoughts. Then thank God for His faithfulness and His promise to give you victory.

 Dear Father, thank You for standing beside me in every battle I face and for winning the victory for all time through Your Son, Jesus Christ.

Heavenly King, give me the strength I need to stand firm in every battle, knowing that You have already defeated the enemy.

DAY 7: *Reflections*

As we close this week, spend some time meditating on the following truths found in Scripture. You may wish to spend this time at your altar.

Lord, you have been our dwelling place throughout all generations. Before the mountains were born or you brought forth the earth and the world, from everlasting to everlasting you are God (Psalm 90:1-2).

[You] satisfy us in the morning with your unfailing love, that we may sing for joy and be glad all our days (Psalm 90:14).

Because I love You and acknowledge Your name, You will rescue me and protect me. I will call upon You and You will answer me; You will be with me in trouble and will deliver and honor me (see Psalm 91:14-15).

Great is our Lord and mighty in power; his understanding has no limit. The LORD sustains the humble (Psalm 147:5-6).

My heart rejoices because I trust in His holy name. May Your unfailing love rest on me, O Lord, as I put my hope in You (see Psalm 33:21-22).

Dear Father, thank You for giving me the authority to overcome every obstacle in my life through prayer, Your Holy Spirit, Your Word and Your limitless love. Thank You for giving me victory through Your Son's sacrifice.

Notes

1. *International Standard Bible Encyclopedia*, vol. 3 (Grand Rapids, MI: William B. Eerdmans Publishing, 1982), s.v. "mustard."
2. James Strong, *The Strongest Strong's Exhaustive Concordance of the Bible* (Grand Rapids, MI: Zondervan Publishing House, 2001), Hebrew #3068.

GROUP PRAYER REQUESTS   TODAY'S DATE:_____

NAME	REQUEST	RESULTS

BEGIN THE PROCESS OF CHANGE

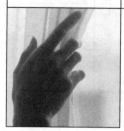

MEMORY VERSE
Let us then approach the throne of grace with confidence, so that we may receive mercy and find grace to help us in our time of need.
Hebrews 4:16

We have learned the importance of desiring and choosing daily to live as new creations in Christ. We have also studied some common obstacles that believers encounter and how to remove those obstacles and experience victory in Christ. Now let's turn our attention to the areas of our lives that need healing and freedom.

Anytime God works in our lives to bring healing and freedom, we are changed or transformed. We become more like Christ. This week we will learn what God's Word teaches us about being transformed and expand on some of the concepts that were introduced earlier in the study.

DAY 1: *Removing the Mask*

Read 2 Corinthians 11:13-15. The word "masquerade" is used three times in these verses. "Masquerade" is derived from the Greek word *metaschmatizo*, which means "to transform, change (the form); to masquerade, disguise oneself."[1]

>> What comes to your mind when you hear the word "masquerade"?

People dressed up, wearing masks
Representing yourself falsely

>> How are Satan and his followers described in these Scriptures?

False teachers, deceitful workers

Why do you think Satan chooses to present himself in this way?

That's the only way he knows.
Any other way we would not obey him.
If we saw him the way he really is.

➤ Based on the descriptions of Satan in 2 Corinthians 11:14 and Genesis 3:1, describe how you think Satan presented himself to Eve.

As an angel of light
falsely

How do you think Satan presents himself to us?

He wiggle in, makes sin look good, doesn't tell the end result.

We will study Genesis 3 in greater detail tomorrow. For today, take a moment to read Genesis 3:1-5.

➤ What did Satan want to do in Eve's life that day in the Garden of Eden?

He want her to doubt God's word and His goodness.

➤ Look back at the definition of "metaschmatizo." According to this definition, who is responsible for making the change, or transformation?

Read Romans 12:2. The word "transformed" is derived from the Greek word *metamorphoo*, which means "to be transformed, transfigured, changed in form."[2] This definition implies there is an outside force making the transformation.

➤ According to Romans 12:2 and the meaning of "metamorphoo," what is responsible for changing, or transforming, our lives?

The Word of God - renewing your mind with

Based on what you have learned in this study, who and what have the power to renew our minds?

God and His Word

Our enemy, Satan, loves the concept of self-help because it convinces people that they can make changes in their lives without God's intervention. We've already discussed the danger of thinking we can do it on our own—the path of pride leads nowhere.

Satan is a counterfeit: His methods are counterfeit and his results are counterfeit. Satan knows that God's Word is powerful and that it will transform a believer's life into the image of God's Son, rather than disguising the same old self as something good.

➤ How does this lesson about transformation apply to your own life?

God is able to transform us, if we let Him

Thank You, Lord, for giving me a brand-new life! Thank You for setting me free from a life of sin and death by transforming my life through Your powerful Word.

Father, I choose to yield my heart to Your commands so that I may grow in the likeness of Your Son. I love and adore You.

DAY 2: *Recognizing Deception*

Today we will continue our study of Genesis 3 to familiarize ourselves with the strategies of our enemy. Read Genesis 3:1-8.

➤ Look closely at Genesis 3:1. What was the first step of Satan's methodical plan to destroy Eve?

Getting her to question God

What was the second step of Satan's plan?

Getting her to doubt God

➤ Compare verses 2 and 3 with Genesis 2:16. What evidence do you find that Satan's plan was working?

Eve was on the defensive

➤ Read Genesis 3:4. What difference do you sense in Satan's tone compared with how he first spoke to Eve in verse 1?

He is no longer suggestive, he was saying God lied.

➤ Notice that in verse 5, Satan switched his focus from what God said to God's character. What do you think Satan was hoping to accomplish?

He want Eve to doubt & diobey God.

John 10:10 says that Satan comes to kill, steal and destroy. We must recognize the enemy's strategies and understand the damage he can do to our lives. Satan's tools include doubting, distorting and disputing God's Word; creating confusion; creating doubt about God's character and distracting us. Read Genesis 3:1-6 again; this time identify how Satan used each of these tools against Eve.

➤ Which of Satan's tools does he use in your life and how does he use them?

Mostly with my thought life. I would never be brave enough to put my thought into practice, thank God!

Have you ever recognized Satan using those tools? Explain.

I have certain convictions. One which is submission to my husband. Through the years as the world has progressed so has the church. Satan has caused me to question some of these convictions, so I won't be an odd ball.

How do you think Satan's tools can affect your ability to live as a new creation in Christ?

He makes me doubt "I can do all things through Christ which strengthens me"

How do you think Satan's tools can affect your ability to accomplish your First Place goals?

Just as Eve did not simply grab the forbidden fruit and start eating it, we do not disobey God without thinking about it first. Like Eve, we entertain a trail of thoughts that leads to each action. Our thoughts either lead us down a path of destruction or a path of victory.

Think of a goal you have set in First Place. Now allow yourself to have several negative, destructive thoughts about meeting that goal. To make matters worse, speak those thoughts aloud. What feelings are surfacing in your heart? Record your thoughts in the space provided.

I am discouraged. I want to quit. It's easier just to do my own thing.

Now think of the same goal and say your memory verse aloud. Think of several other Scriptures that encourage you to stay on track. Thank God for the wonderful things He is doing in your life and for the victory He has and will continue to give you. How do you feel now? Record your thoughts in the space provided.

I feel renewed, ready to go out there and win, accompolish my goals

Thank You, O Lord, that Your Word transforms my life! Your Word is more powerful than any of Satan's tools.

Teach me, Father, to be transformed by the renewing of my mind [see Romans 12:2]. I want to be more like Christ and experience greater healing and freedom in my life.

DAY 3: *Marching to Battle*

We learned yesterday that Satan's tools include doubting, distorting and disputing God's Word; creating confusion; creating doubt about God's character and distracting us. Bottom line, Satan's tools are designed to build deception in our lives.

➤ According to 2 Corinthians 11:3, how might we be led astray from our sincere and pure devotion to Christ?

Being deceived by satan's cunning

"Sincere and pure devotion" in this verse is derived from the Greek word *haplotes*, which means "singleness; sincerity."[3] In other words, we are to be sincere and have a singleness of purpose and motivation.

➤ What do you think it means to be sincere and to have a singleness of purpose and motivation in regard to your relationship with Christ?

Put it first, guard it, work at it, really want it

Ps. 94:11
The Lord
k. the
thoughts
of man,

What do you think it means to have a singleness of purpose and motivation in your thought life?

Phil 2:5

Same! read and memorize the Word. Guard (keep watch on) your thoughts.

Let this be mind be in you

Isa. 55:8
My t.
are not
your t.

The phrase "led astray" in this verse is derived from a Greek word we studied in week one: "phtheiro." "Phtheiro" means "to destroy by means of corrupting."

☞ What does the definition of "phtheiro" teach us about the danger of not being sincere, of lacking a singleness of purpose and motivation in our thought life?

Corruption can set in.

Let's try to gain a clearer perspective of how our enemy works. Second Corinthians 11:3 says that Eve "was deceived by the serpent's cunning." Some synonyms for "deception" include "fraud" and "trickery."[4] Synonyms for "cunning" include "subtlety," "craftiness" and "cleverness."[5]

☞ Using your understanding of the words "deception" and "cunning," describe how Satan works in our lives.

He doesn't hit us full on w/ temptation, he comes softly, a little at a time, worming his way a little at a time.

☞ Summarize what you have learned through the study of 2 Corinthians 11:3 concerning the battle of your mind.

Keep your mind stayed on Christ, lest we be tricked by satan. I believe sin is conceived in the mind before

What have you learned about the importance of your thought life?

Guard it, moniter it, protect it.

Praise be to You, Father of my Lord Jesus Christ, who has blessed me in the heavenly realms with every spiritual blessing in Christ. Thank You for choosing me in Him before the creation of the world to be holy and blameless in Your sight [see Ephesians 1:3-4].

Father, I celebrate today the new life You have given me. Help me to guard my thoughts against Satan's craftiness and deception so that I can live as a new creation in Christ.

DAY 4: *Waging War*

As we have discovered, the battle with our enemy begins in our thought life. When we follow God's instructions as outlined in His Word, we are guaranteed victory; however, we must allow God to reveal the enemy's tools and how he uses them in our lives.

Read 2 Corinthians 10:3-5. These verses teach us how to fight a spiritual battle—a battle between God's soldiers and our enemy, Satan.

➤ What do you think it means to wage war or to serve as a soldier in a spiritual battle?

We are constantly defending our selves against satan in our mind. If we are spiritually mined re: the battle

Just as in a military battle between two opposing parties, the leadership of our spiritual battle plays a vital role in the outcome.

➤ What does Colossians 2:9-10 tell us about the leadership of both armies in the battle we are fighting?

We are complete in Him, who is the Head of all powers & authorities

➤ Reread 2 Corinthians 10:4. Based on what you have learned in this study, what weapons do we use for battle?

God's power, read & memorize the Word.   Christ used this in His temptation

➤ According to 2 Corinthians 10:4-5, what do the weapons we use attack?

strongholds - arguments & every pretension that sets itself up against the knowledge of God.

A stronghold can be either a fortress or a prison.[6] In this verse, a stronghold is an almost impenetrable prison.

⤳ Briefly describe what you think a prison would be like for a soldier who had been captured in a battle.

I can't imagine. I know some of our soldiers were not treated very well. You're at the command of the enemy.

If a soldier had been fighting the battle alone, how difficult do you think it would be to escape that prison?

Probably impossible

In our study of Genesis 3, we identified several tools of the enemy: doubting, distorting and disputing God's Word; creating confusion; creating doubt in God's character and distracting us.

⤳ Which of these tools can be defeated by the weapons described in 2 Corinthians 10:3-5?

All these

⤳ Give an example of an argument that contradicts what you know to be true about God.

God doen't care about me, He's up there in heaven
away

⤳ How can prideful or pretentious thoughts battle against the knowledge of God?

The battle is fought in the mind. The Holy Spirit helps us have the mind of Christ.

Remember, Satan is a counterfeit. He disguises himself as something good and pleasing. As with Eve, Satan uses his pretentious nature to deceive us.

⤳ Read 2 Corinthians 10:5 again. What do you think to "take captive every thought and to make it obedient to Christ" means?

Keep your thought life in check w/ memorizing the Word, thinking on Christ + others.

>> How will your thoughts influence your success in First Place?

Every victory gives confidence. You can do it.

Experiencing victory on the battlefield of our minds is a significant part of living as new creations in Christ. Though nothing can ever take away our identity as new creations, we must choose to believe and walk in the truth of God's Word to experience true victory and freedom in our lives.

Thank You, Father, for continually transforming me into a greater likeness of Your beloved Son. Lord, I surrender my thought life to You. I want my mind to be renewed by Your powerful Word.

God, thank You that Your Word destroys the work of the enemy. I praise You and declare that You are King of kings and Lord of lords.

DAY 5: *Walking in the Light*

Yesterday we briefly discussed the word "stronghold." We learned that a stronghold can be either a fortress or a prison. A stronghold is something built to surround a person, either to protect the person or to keep him or her from escaping. As we have learned, Satan uses his set of tools to try to build strongholds in our lives that will hold us captive.

>> Based on what you have learned about a stronghold and what you have learned about Satan's tools, how is a stronghold built in a person's thought life?

Satan tools can hold you prisoner OR Christ can protect you from him.

How do you think sin can become a stronghold in a person's life?

When sin holds dominion over you, you are a prisoner

❧ According to Luke 4:18-19, what did Jesus come to do for the prisoners, the blind and the oppressed?

To set them free.

Have you ever felt like a prisoner? Blind? Oppressed? Explain.

I think all women, maybe men too, at times feel prisoners to their commitments. I love what I do, but there are times

Remember, our identity can never be taken from us. We have been given new life in Christ and have been declared free. However, old patterns of thinking, strongholds, sin, unforgiveness and unhealed hurts can make us feel the pain and agony of bondage.

❧ Read Ephesians 5:8-11. What instructions are we given (vv. 8-10)?

Live as children of light in goodness, righteousness & truth. Find out what pleases the Lord Shun & expose fruitless deeds of darkness

What does God want us to do with the deeds, or works, of darkness (v. 11)?

❧ Read Ephesians 5:13-14. How are the deeds of darkness—the enemy's handiwork—in our lives revealed?

By the Light of God's Word

❧ How is God described in 1 John 1:5?

God is Light

⇛ Read John 14:16-17. How does Jesus describe the Holy Spirit in these verses?

Comforter, Spirit of truth

⇛ According to John 16:13, to where does the Holy Spirit guide us?

into all truth

⇛ Write 3 John 1:4 in the space provided.

"I have no greater joy than to hear that my children walk in truth."

⇛ In summary, what do the verses we read today tell us about walking in truth versus walking in darkness?

God is pleased with us & we are happier.

⇛ Based on 1 Peter 2:9, describe your identity and your purpose.

We are a chosen generation, a royal priesthood, an holy people, peculiar people, we should praise God, who called us out of darkness into His marvelous Light.

Father, thank You for wanting to reveal Yourself to me in a greater way. You desire to bring healing and freedom to every part of my heart and mind.

Lord, prepare me for the work that You want to do in my life. You are the potter and I am the clay. I choose to entrust myself fully to the hands of my maker.

DAY 6: *Reflections*

This week we learned that a stronghold is a prison that is built to surround an individual so that he or she cannot escape. We also learned that we have been given God's Word, prayer and the Holy Spirit as weapons to destroy strongholds.

Satan is a counterfeit who masquerades as an angel of light. He uses his set of tools to deceive us and lead us astray. He attempts to build strongholds in our lives to keep us imprisoned by a belief system built on his lies or by our own sin.

Remember that the word "stronghold" can also mean "a fortress." Psalm 18:2 says, "The LORD is my rock, my fortress and my deliverer; my God is my rock, in whom I take refuge. He is my shield and the horn of my salvation, my stronghold." God wants us to see Him as our deliverer who provides a place where our hearts can find peace and rest from the storms of life. God encamps around us, a mighty fortress built by His Son's nail-scarred hands. The walls are built with grace and truth. Freedom echoes throughout the spacious palace. We are welcomed every time we visit. We were created to make it our home.

The strongholds Satan builds lack the authority and power to keep prisoners from finding freedom. However, the stronghold built by the nail-scarred hands of Jesus will last for all eternity. Praise God!

Dear Father, thank You for being my fortress and my deliverer. I desire to take refuge in You, to escape the attacks of the enemy. Only in You will I find complete safety and peace.

DAY 7: *Reflections*

The Bible describes God's throne as a throne of grace. God is King of kings and Lord of lords; His throne is far above any powers or authorities, and His reign lasts forever. Yet this mighty God describes His throne as a throne of *grace*. Grace is God's favor, undeservedly yet freely bestowed on us. God tells us to enter His throne room with confidence as His Son declares that we are members of the royal family.

Consider what we have learned in our study about becoming new creations. Because of the Lord's passion for us, He has provided a way for us to dwell at God's throne of grace. However, feelings of condemnation, doubt and fear can keep us from entering that throne room. How can God receive the glory He deserves when His children are too insecure to approach their Father in heaven with confidence?

The confidence we are to embrace as we enter the throne room of God comes from knowing and believing that we have died to our old selves and that our lives are now hidden with Christ (see Colossians 3:3). Jesus' blood now covers us and makes us holy and blameless in God's sight (see Ephesians 1:4).

Spend a few moments in prayer at your altar. Consider what you have learned this week about the process of being transformed by God's Word.

Heavenly Father, I come to Your throne room with confidence, knowing that I stand before You covered by the cleansing power of Jesus' blood.

Thank You, great King, for making me a part of Your royal family. I am so privileged to be called Your child.

Notes

1. James Strong, *The Strongest Strong's Exhaustive Concordance of the Bible* (Grand Rapids, MI: Zondervan Publishing House, 2001), Greek #3345.
2. Ibid., Greek #3339.
3. Ibid., Greek #572.
4. *Merriam-Webster's Collegiate Dictionary*, 11th ed., s.v. "deception."
5. *The New Roget's Thesaurus*, rev. ed., s.v. "cunning."
6. Strong, *The Strongest Strong's Exhaustive Concordance of the Bible*, Greek #3794.

GROUP PRAYER REQUESTS TODAY'S DATE:_____

NAME	REQUEST	RESULTS
Young Family Gothards	death	
Hayes Family	death	
Pursoo	Stomach cancer	
Kelly	quit smoking	
Lampkey	death	
Donna	mary's sister	

THE HEART OF GOD

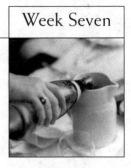

MEMORY VERSE
*For we are God's workmanship, created
in Christ Jesus to do good works, which
God prepared in advance for us to do.*
Ephesians 2:10

God desires His children to know truth and to walk in it. Last week we learned that our enemy wants us to travel a different path—a path wrought with deception. This week we will continue to discover God's heart and dispel any misconceptions we may have about Him. Having a clear understanding of God's heart will allow us to readily trust Him with ours.

DAY 1: *Beginning the Journey*

Our earthly fathers have a significant influence on how we perceive our heavenly Father. Today's lesson may be sensitive—even painful—for some of us; however, we need to recognize how our earthly fathers have influenced our beliefs about our heavenly Father and allow God's Word to change any distorted beliefs we may have about Him.

➽ Read Romans 12:2. For review, explain how we are transformed.

by the renewing of our mind

According to this verse, what is one of the benefits of changing our thought and belief system?

to be able to test and approve what God's will is - His good, pleasing and perfect will

How does this concept apply to our thoughts and beliefs about God?

God loves us. His will for us reflects that.

➤ Read Psalm 139:23-24. Why do you think we need God's help to know our hearts and our anxious thoughts?

We are not always honest with ourself. We make excuses.

➤ What do you think it means to have an "offensive way" (v. 24) in us?

unconfessed sin

Based on what we learned last week, what is the origin of offensive or wicked ways?

Satan

Our thoughts either lead us down a road paved with truth or a road paved with deception. The road we decide to travel will play a key role in forming our beliefs—beliefs either based on God's truth or based on Satan's lies.

➤ How do you think Satan uses painful life experiences as opportunities to introduce lies?

He wants us to doubt God's love and care of us.

Why do you think our painful experiences are ideal times for those lies to develop from thoughts into belief systems?

That's when we are more vulerable

➤ How do you think painful experiences with our earthly fathers can pave a road in our thoughts and beliefs that leads us away from experiencing intimacy with our heavenly Father?

We may be leary about trusting our heavenly Father, since our earthly father failed us.

How do you think your childhood experiences with your earthly father set a precedent for your journey in life with your heavenly Father?

If I depended on those experiences I would NEVER trust my HEAVENLY Father. God has healed me, I rarely question Him today.

Read Romans 8:38-39. How would you use this verse to encourage someone who has been severely hurt by his or her earthly father?

NOTHING can seperate me from God's love.

Based on what you have learned in this study about God's character, list several truths about your heavenly Father that show His faithfulness, goodness, perfection and His love for you.

Heavenly Father, Your love is more powerful than any pain I have or will ever experience in life. The power of Your love sets me free from a life of sin and death.

Father, I want to be consumed by Your love. Begin removing the obstacles in my heart and mind that prevent me from experiencing the tremendous depth of Your love.

DAY 2: *Dispelling Misconceptions*

Throughout Scripture God has displayed His passion for leading His people down the road to freedom. One of God's greatest joys is knowing that His beloved children are walking on the path paved by truth. God is jealous for us to enter into His presence with a solid understanding of His amazing love for us.

➤ Why do you think misconceptions about God can affect our ability to enter into an intimate and tender relationship with Him?

Know the truth, it will set you free

To Know the truth about God gives you the freedom & trust to have this relationship

In 2 Corinthians 4:2, Paul gives us several instructions for handling God's Word. Read the verse, and then answer the following questions.

➤ What do you think it means to renounce "secret and shameful ways," and what benefit do we receive when we do so?

Acts we do that we think ~~only~~ Noone knows about, but God Knows all things. maybe thoughts, how we feel about our brothers & sister in Christ. Confess all = Clear conscience

➤ What do you think it means to "use deception," and how can we avoid using it in our own lives? *maybe hypocrisy - false front Telling only half truths that leads to false conclusions*

➤ How do you think we might "distort the word of God" in our own thought life? *Justifing what we want to do, even though the principles of the Word say nay.*

➤ How can we set forth the truth plainly? *Living Godly & righteously before God & man*

Secret and shameful ways encompass a lot of things, including sinful thoughts and behaviors, shameful thoughts and habits, and even feelings of deep shame because of another's sin that has damaged us.

For this lesson we will concentrate on how 2 Corinthians 4:2 applies to our thought life.

⇛ What do you think it means to renounce secret and shameful thoughts? *Confess them to God, don't dwell on them. Get some Scripture to memorize, get your mind elsewhere. TRy to figure the end result.*

Secrets are things that are not disclosed. Secret thoughts are thoughts that are somehow hidden. We have learned that a belief system begins with a simple thought. When the enemy lies to us through a thought and we do not cast it away, but allow it to remain at home in our minds, the thought will eventually become a belief. *or sin.*

⇛ Based on what you have learned through the study of God's Word, can we have a belief system that is hidden, or secret, even to us? *Yes*

Psalm 44:21 tells us that God "knows the secrets of the heart." God is all knowing and nothing is hidden from Him. God has also given us the Counselor, His Holy Spirit, to guide us into His truth (see John 16:13). As you remember from last week's study, the deeds of darkness in our lives are exposed by the light, and "God is light; in Him there is no darkness at all" (1 John 1:5; see also Ephesians 5:13-14).

⇛ Review Psalm 139:23-24. Why do you think your heavenly Father wants you to ask Him to search your deepest parts and to bring into the light anything offensive?

Only then can we walk in truth and know the peace & joy of walking in His will.

Our heavenly Father knows that when our beliefs about Him are formed using the truth of God's Word, we will run across the threshold into His loving presence. We will seek Him with passion and joy.

⇛ How do you think entering into God's presence would affect your daily relationship with Him?

It's like walking into your home and shutting the door & shutting the world out. You are safe & secure. You trust Him totally. think about having this every day.

Praise the Lord.!

How would it affect your ability to meet your goals in First Place?

To be totally honest about all things, + have Him help me w/this - I will have success.

Thank You, God, for setting me apart for Yourself and that You will hear me when I call to You [see Psalm 4:3].

Father, I ask You to search my deepest parts and bring into Your light any offensive thing in me. I desire to walk across the threshold into Your loving presence.

DAY 3: *Revealing Secrets*

We know that God is jealous for us and that He sent Jesus so that we can live in freedom. God can heal the deepest wounds and break the thickest chains of bondage; however, God's healing and freedom occur in the light. Only in the light can truth be distinguished from deception and sin be clearly seen. Only in the light can the wounds of our hearts finally be mended.

Today we will concentrate on identifying any thoughts and beliefs that we have about God that are based on Satan's lies.

➤ For review, what tools did Satan use against Eve?

deception - question + doubt God pride

What was the purpose of Satan's encounter with Eve?

To get her to disobey God

➤ Why can deception cause tremendous damage in our relationship with God?

We don't have the freedom to walk + talk w/ Him

➤ Read James 1:5. What do we need to do to gain wisdom?

Ask

Why do you think we need God's wisdom to identify deception in our lives?

We don't always want to admit it is deception.

Grab a pen and a piece of paper or your journal and head to your special altar. Take a few moments to ask God to prepare you for what He wants to do in your life through this study. Share any fears, concerns or doubts you may have. Ask God to give you His peace and strength, and the wisdom you need to recognize any deception in your life.

Now ask God to reveal to you the following: (1) any lies that you believe about Him, (2) any lies that you believe about God's love for you and (3) any lies that you believe about your relationship with Him. You may use the following prayer or your own words. On the piece of paper or in your journal, write down everything that God puts on your heart.

Father, I ask You to search my heart and my thoughts. Reveal any lies from the enemy that I believe. God, expose all deception by shining Your light into the dark places of my heart and mind.

Father, I ask You to reveal any lies that I believe about You or Your love for me.

Father, please reveal any lies that I believe about my relationship with You.

Thank You, Father, for revealing these lies to me. Thank You that the work of the enemy has been exposed by the power of Your love for me. Continue the process of setting me free from the pain of deception. I commit my mind and my heart fully to You. In Jesus' name, amen.

Note: Do not be discouraged if you did not hear clearly from God. Praying in this way may be new to you. You may want to call someone in your group or a First Place leader and ask him or her to pray with you. Remember, part of being in First Place is growing in your relationship with God through the help of other believers.

➤ Based on the lies that God revealed to you today, why do you think a wrong belief about God can cause us pain?

> *Years of not having that closeness, peace & joy can cause physical, mental and spiritual problems*

➤ How do you think the lies that you believed about God and His love have affected your relationship with Him?

> *They keep us from coming to Him freely w/ every problem & concern.*

➤ Can you see any way that the enemy may have used wounds caused by your earthly father as an opportunity to introduce his lies? Explain.

> *At one time I did, but God has opened my eyes. My heavely Father is NOTHING like my earthly father*

We know that God's Word has the power to destroy the strongest lies and transform our lives. Tomorrow we will learn how to replace our wrong beliefs with truth so that we can experience freedom from the bondage of deception.

Thank You, God, for setting me free to walk in complete truth. I know that You are doing a work in my life and that You will be faithful to complete it [see Philippians 1:6].

DAY 4: *Restoring Truth*

It is God's desire and will for our lives that we know and believe His Word. God wants us to see ourselves and our lives the way He sees them.

➤ Read each of the following verses. In the space provided, note how God's Word describes you.

Psalm 139:14

> *I am fearfully & wonderfully made*

Isaiah 64:8

I am the work of His hands

2 Corinthians 5:17

I am a new creation

Galatians 3:27

I am clothed w/ CHRIST

Galatians 4:6-7

I am a son & heir

Ephesians 1:4-5

I am holy & blameless in His sight

Ephesians 3:12

I can call on God w/ freedom & confidence

➤ Read each of the following verses. In the space provided, note what God's Word says about God's love for you.

Psalm 103:17

It is everlasting

Jeremiah 31:3

It is everlasting

Lamentations 3:22-23

It is a great love

John 3:16

God so loved, He gave

Romans 8:38-39

Nothing can separate us His love

➤ Read Hebrews 4:12. How is God's Word "living and active" in our lives?

It judges the thoughts & intents of the heart.

How do you think God's Word penetrates to the deepest parts of our hearts and lives?

When we read & study, the Holy Spirit gives us the sincere desire to measure up

How do you think God's Word judges the thoughts and attitudes of our hearts?

It is a measure to help us judge ourself

According to Isaiah 55:10-11, what does God's Word do in our lives?

It accompolishes what God desires + achieves the purpose for which He sent it.

Read the following verses. In the space provided, note what each verse says about God's Word.

Deuteronomy 8:3

Man shall not live by bread alone but by every word that comes

Psalm 119:11

Thy Word have I hid in my heart, that I might not sin against God

Psalm 119:105

How sweet are your words to my mouth, sweeter than honey

John 1:1-2

Jesus was The Word.

Read Matthew 4:1-11. How did Jesus respond to Satan's attack?

With the Word

Based on the Scriptures you have read today, how can you restore truth to your heart and mind?

By spending time in the Word

Remember, Jesus Christ gives us our identity as new creations at the moment of salvation. However, old thought patterns and belief systems can rob us of the joy, peace and freedom that God desires His children to enjoy. Praise God that His Word is working in our lives to demolish those defeating thoughts and belief systems! Let's walk in His truth and live our lives free of deception.

 Father God, I praise You that Your Word is working in my life to demolish defeating thoughts and belief systems. Please give me the wisdom and strength I need to walk in truth and to live my life free of deception.

DAY 5: *Believing God's Word*

The title of our study this week is "The Heart of God." So far, we have learned that our earthly fathers impact our relationship with God. We asked God to reveal how the enemy's tools of deception have skewed our thoughts and beliefs about God. Yesterday we examined Scriptures to discover the immense power God's Word can have on our lives. Today we will learn how to experience freedom from deception by replacing lies with truth.

On Day 3 of this week you asked God to reveal any lies that you believed about Him, His love for you and your relationship with Him. You then wrote down what God put on your heart. Please look at the list of lies that God revealed to you.

Draw a line down the center of a blank sheet of paper. Write the word "Lies" on the top left side of the page and the word "Truth" on the top right side of the page. List each lie that God revealed to you under the column titled "Lies."

For each lie listed in the left-hand column, choose a Scripture to replace the lie. Write each Scripture in the column titled "Truth" across from the corresponding lie. You may choose a verse we studied on Day 4, or God may bring a special verse to mind. Follow the Holy Spirit's leading.

Take this list to your altar. Second Corinthians 4:2 tells us to renounce "secret and shameful ways." "Renounce" means "to give up; to refuse to follow, obey, or recognize further."[1] God has revealed secret thoughts and beliefs that are based on lies. The next step is simply to refuse to follow those lies. Pray and renounce each individual lie aloud. You may use the prayer below or your own words.

> *In the name of Jesus Christ, I renounce the lie that [insert lie]. I refuse to believe this lie any longer. Thank You, Jesus, for exposing this as a lie from the enemy. I ask You to remove the power that this lie has had on my life. Thank You, Jesus, that You came to set me free. Forgive me for believing this lie. I now choose to reject, disown and abandon it. Thank You, Jesus, that I am free from the power this lie has had on my life. In Your precious name, amen.*

Once a lie has been exposed, it loses the power it had to cause us to stumble around in the dark. By bringing all our thoughts into the light, we can see lies for what they really are and we can replace them with God's truth.

➤ Why is it important to be attentive to your thoughts?

They motivate you actions

➤ When you recognize a thought as being false, what should you immediately choose to do with that thought?

Try to replace it with a verse of Scripture

What is the next thing that you must do to completely destroy the lie and change your mind-set?

Pray + renounce it out loud Write it down

The discipline of rejecting lies and replacing them with God's Word will transform our lives (see Romans 12:2). It is a discipline that we need to practice daily to live as new creations in Christ.

➤ Why do you think this discipline needs to be practiced daily?

To prevent these thoughts + lies from taking root

How do you think this discipline applies to keeping the Nine Commitments of First Place?

A disciplined life leads to sucess.

➤ Look at the column of lies and the column of truths you created earlier. How will you apply the discipline of replacing lies with truth the next time the enemy fires one of those lies in your direction?

Write it down, pray + renouce it out loud.

Father, I ask You to give me wisdom and understanding, for they are more profitable than silver and yield better returns that gold [see Proverbs 3:13-14].

Lord, create in me a heart that seeks You and a passion to know Your Word. I desire to walk in Your truth.

DAY 6: *Reflections*

Learning to live as new creations in Christ and allowing God to transform our lives are exciting journeys. For some, it may feel a little scary. The familiar sometimes feels more comfortable and safe than an adventure into the unknown.

God tells us that we are His "workmanship" (Ephesians 2:10). This word is derived from the Greek word *poiema*, from which we derive the English word "poem."[2] We are God's poems, and our author is a skilled writer. He knows how every line will work together to create a masterpiece that will be beautiful to its readers and bring praise to the writer.

Take a few moments and allow God to lavish His love on you. Tell God that you want Him to draw your heart close to His. Tell God that you want Him and that you need Him. Believe that God's Word is true, and allow the Scriptures we studied this week to drown out any fears or condemning thoughts. Now sit at His feet until you are pouring your love back to Him.

Father, thank You for turning my life into a beautiful master-piece. May every line of my life bring praise and glory to You.

Lord, thank You for loving me with reckless abandon. May my heart grow to return Your love more each day.

DAY 7: *Reflections*

Once upon a time there was a man—not just an ordinary man, mind you, but a man born with an extraordinary heart. His parents knew from the start that their son was born with a destiny that was beyond their under-standing. As the child grew and became a man, the world around him was frightened and confused by the man's plan. How could a man give sight to the blind and heal the sick? How could a man calm the raging sea and silence the enemy? How could a man offer salvation—an eternity with God? How could a man rescue the oppressed and give them liberty? How could a man fill a heart abundantly and change a life so beautifully? This man could, because His name was Jesus.

The heart of God is most easily seen in the life of His beloved Son, Jesus, who reflects the passion, the grace and the compelling love of His beloved Father. No matter what kind of start you have had in life, no mat-ter what kind of foundation you are trying to stand on and no matter what kinds of secrets you are harboring, God passionately wants you to walk in His truth and freedom. The heart of God was crucified on a cross so that you could know Him. That is the heart of God.

Dear Father, once again my heart is overwhelmed by the life of one man: Your beloved Son. Thank You for sending Him to Earth to bring freedom and healing to the captives. I am a new creation because of His life, death and resurrection.

Notes

1. *Merriam-Webster's Collegiate Dictionary*, 11th ed., s.v. "renounce."
2. James Strong, *The Strongest Strong's Exhaustive Concordance of the Bible* (Grand Rapids, MI: Zondervan Publishing House, 2001), Greek #4161.

GROUP PRAYER REQUESTS TODAY'S DATE:_____

NAME	REQUEST	RESULTS
Strohs	car accident	
Thompson		
Harry *Gladys* Spurlock	Teresa parents	
Rachel		
Johnson	Stomach cancer	
diana + *Jim*	aaron's sister	
Jon Perry	Cal.	

FIND HEALING FOR YOUR HEART

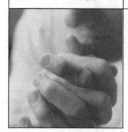

MEMORY VERSE

The LORD your God is with you, he is mighty to save.
He will take great delight in you, he will quiet you
with his love, he will rejoice over you with singing.

Zephaniah 3:17

We have learned that deceptive thoughts are destructive and create feelings of hopelessness, helplessness and despair. Those destructive thoughts hinder us from living as new creations in Christ. We have also learned that God's Word has the power to destroy those destructive thoughts and that we are transformed when we replace destructive thoughts with God's Word.

Another hindrance to living as new creations in Christ is a wounded heart. Heart wounds are life experiences that have caused us deep pain. When these wounds are left unhealed, the pain in our hearts prevents us from experiencing the joy that marks new creations in Christ. This week we will identify steps that we can take in our lives to bring healing to our heart wounds.

DAY 1: *Accepting Healing*

Today we will discover through Scripture the healing power of our Lord and Savior, Jesus Christ.

➤ Read Matthew 4:24 and 15:30. List the wounds that Jesus healed.

Various deseases
severe pain
demon, possession
seizures

paralyzed
lame, blind, crippled
mute

➤ Read Mark 10:51-52. What did this man possess that affected his healing?

faith

➣ Read Matthew 9:20-22. What did this woman possess that affected her healing?

faith

➣ According to 1 John 5:1,5, what are the products of our belief in God?

Belief in Jesus, His Son
Overcoming the World

➣ Read Hebrews 11:6. Describe the significance of our faith.

Without faith it is impossible to please God

➣ According to Ephesians 6:16, how is our faith used against the attacks of the enemy?

It helps us quench all the fiery darts of the wicked

➣ How do you think faith in God, in His Word and in His ability to heal heart wounds can affect our healing? How can lack of faith?

According to Scripture, faith in Christ will heal; but without Him we can do nothing.

➣ What are your thoughts and feelings regarding God's willingness and ability to heal the wounds of your heart?

I know God heals, I have experienced it many times.

➣ Have you ever considered that overeating may be a response to pain from a wound that has not been healed? Do you believe this may be true of you? Explain.

No. I just love to cook and I love to eat.

➤ Read Psalm 147:3 and Isaiah 61:1. What does Jesus desire to do in your life?

Heal us and set us free

➤ What does Isaiah 53:4-5 tell you about your wounds?

By His wounds we are healed

Close today's lesson by sharing your heart with God. Tell Him any concerns or doubts you have about His desire to heal your heart wounds. Thank Jesus for the pain and death He suffered so that you could experience healing. Write your prayer in the space provided or in your journal.

II Kings 5 Naaman

DAY 2: *Trusting God*

The first step in healing a wounded heart is trusting God. Choosing to trust God with our hearts can be an extremely difficult decision to make. If our earthly fathers or people we have trusted have damaged our hearts, we will have more difficulty trusting our heavenly Father. If we have believed many lies about God and His love for us, we will also have a more difficult time trusting God with our hearts.

➤ Why do you think trusting God is the first step in healing?

Trusting anyone can lead to healing, why not God, He will never let you down

⇨ How do you feel about trusting God to heal any wounds in your heart?

He has healed many wounds for me

⇨ Read Proverbs 3:5. Have you ever considered it a sin to refuse to trust God and to instead depend on your own understanding? Why or why not?

This is my life verse. Yes, I think it's a sin. How could we not, He loved me and died for me, He wants us to love & trust Him.

⇨ According to Psalm 28:7, what happens when we trust God with our hearts?

We are helped

⇨ Read Psalm 84:12. What happens when we trust God?

We are blessed

⇨ According to John 14:1, what does Jesus ask us to do with our hearts?

Let them not be troubled

Trusting God with our hearts is something we must choose to do. Take a moment to write a prayer to God in the space provided or in your journal. Tell God any fears you may have and ask Him to give you His peace. Make a decision to trust God with your heart.

Dear Lord,
I think I do trust you w/ my whole heart. If not, then search me, & know my thoughts. Reveal to me any doubts I may have about trusting you.

Last week we learned the importance of believing truth and rejecting lies. We have learned that one of the enemy's tools is deception. Deception often operates in the secret, or hidden, places of our lives. We know that Jesus exposes the deeds of darkness so that we can walk in the light of His truth. Satan wants God's children to remain in bondage and never experience the healing of Jesus Christ.

≫ Based on what you have learned, how do you think the enemy will try to sabotage your decision to trust God with your heart?

By keeping you too busy to spend time w/ Him.

≫ How do you think the enemy might work in your life to prevent your heart from experiencing healing from painful wounds?

Keep bringing them up.

The healing power of Jesus is powerful and effective. When Jesus heals our wounds, we are truly healed. The world teaches us to cover up our wounds and to walk around ignoring or masking the pain.

≫ What are some ways that you have attempted to ignore or hide the pain from the wounds you have experienced?

Not admitting them out loud

We need to ask God to show us any lies we believe about trusting Him and about our healing. With a blank piece of paper and a pen, go to your special place to meet with God. Draw a line down the center of your paper and label the left-hand side "Lies" and the right-hand side "Truths."

Ask God to reveal any lies that prevent you from trusting Him with your heart; then ask Him to reveal any lies that you believe about Jesus' ability to heal the wounds you've been harboring. You can modify the prayer provided in Day 3 of last week's lesson or use your own words. Remember to pray aloud.

In the left-hand column, write the lies God revealed to you. Renounce or reject these lies. Then, in the right-hand column, replace each lie with a verse that you studied today or any specific Scripture God brings to mind. Tell God that you are choosing to believe His Word and trust Him.

Father, I know that my heart is safe with You and that I can trust You to heal the painful wounds I have been harboring. Thank You for giving me Your Word so that I can learn these truths.

DAY 3: *Revealing Wounds*

Last week we discovered that the Lord knows our hearts and that we can trust Him. The Lord knows every wound we have ever experienced, every tear that we have cried and every tear that we have fought back. He knows which wounds have been healed by His grace and which wounds we have forbidden Him to touch.

⟫ In what ways do you think we refuse God access to some wounds?

Maybe deep wounds, we don't admit to ourselves. Maybe we don't trust Him enough to heal them.

⟫ Why do you think we allow God access to some wounds and not to others?

Maybe we like nursing those wounds, they have been w/us so long, they are like companions.

We don't need to analyze or guess when it comes to our hearts. There is a much better way. We simply need to ask God to show us any wounds that need His healing. Some of us may have only one or two wounds that need healing. Others may have a long list of hurts that God wants to heal. Similarly, the time it takes to heal varies from person to person. God knows what He desires to accomplish in our lives during our journey to healing and freedom.

Take a pen and a piece of paper or your journal and go to your altar. You may use the following prayer or your own words. Write down what God places on your heart.

> *Father, I choose to give You my heart. I trust that the work You are doing in my life is for my good and for Your glory. I believe that You sent Jesus to heal my heart and set me free. I want to receive complete healing from any wounds that are keeping me in pain and bondage. I ask You to reveal any wounds that You want to heal in my life. In the name of Jesus, amen.*

Often, other people are responsible for inflicting our deepest wounds. A huge part of our healing is forgiving those who have hurt us. Unforgiveness is a wound that we inflict on ourselves.

> What painful and harmful emotions do you think exist in a heart that harbors unforgiveness?

Plots to get even
Persecution complex
Occupies your mind w/bad thoughts

> According to Matthew 6:14-15, what is the consequence of unforgiveness?

Unforgiveness from the Father

Forgiveness is a choice. We choose to forgive or choose to harbor unforgiveness. Some wounds inflicted by people in our lives are absolutely impossible for us to forgive using our own strength.

Forgiveness may be extremely difficult, but it is always possible. Through the death and resurrection of Jesus Christ, forgiveness is a finished work. As new creations in Christ we have the power of the Holy Spirit in us, which enables us to forgive.

Using the following prayer or your own words, ask God to reveal anyone that you need to forgive. On a piece of paper or in your journal, write down any names that God places on your heart.

> *Father, search me and know my heart. Bring to light any offensive way in me and lead me in Your everlasting way [see Psalm 139:23-24]. Lord, I want to be completely healed and freed from the wound of unforgiveness. Reveal to me anyone whom I need to forgive. In Jesus' name, amen.*

Today's lesson may have caused painful emotions to surface. Your feelings are not a surprise to God. You have been carrying them behind closed doors in your heart, but it is time to receive healing. When you feel tempted to mask the pain with overeating, tell God how you are feeling and ask Him to give you strength and hope. In those moments, you may want to spend a little time reading through your favorite psalms.

Father, You are my King and I trust You. I will not rely on my own understanding, but trust in You at all times. Thank You for making my paths straight as I acknowledge You in all my ways [see Proverbs 3:5-6].

DAY 4: Breaking the Chain of Unforgiveness

Unforgiveness can wrap around our hearts and keep us in incredible bondage. It can lead to depression, anxiety, fear and bitterness, and it robs us of the joy, peace and freedom that God desires for us.

➤ Read Ephesians 4:32 and fill in the blanks:

Be kind and compassionate to one another, _forgiving_ each other, just as ~~Christ~~ _Christ_ _as in_ God _forgave_ you.

Why do you think God reminded these people of the forgiveness they had received?

If we are forgiven, shouldn't we also be able to forgive.

➤ In Colossians 3:13, what are we asked to do?

Bear w/ each other + forgive whatever grievances you may have against one another. Forgive as the Lord forgave you.

How are we supposed to do this?

With God's help

➤ In Matthew 9:1-8, Jesus healed a paralyzed man. However, Jesus made it clear that He had performed a greater miracle in the man's life. What was that miracle?

He forgave his sins

What does this passage teach us about forgiveness?

It is more important to be forgiven than to be made well.

➳ Yesterday we asked God to show us people whom we need to forgive. Based on the Scriptures you read today, how do we forgive people?

With the help of the Holy Spirit, remembering what Christ did for us.

That the death and resurrection of Jesus Christ covers the sins of the whole world is nothing short of a miracle. Since we have received such an extravagant gift of grace in our own lives, and since we have received the Holy Spirit to transform our hearts, we are enabled to forgive others, no matter what offense they have committed against us. Remember, God forgave the worst sin imaginable: the murder of His Son.

If we are to experience complete freedom, we cannot harbor unforgiveness toward anyone. The enemy will lie and tell us that forgiving someone means that we are denying what the person did or saying that what he or she did was okay. On the contrary, when we choose to forgive someone, we are surrendering our right to judge and condemn and releasing to Christ the anger, bitterness and pain that have kept our hearts in bondage. Forgiveness sets our hearts free!

You can use this closing prayer when forgiving people on your list or anyone who sins against you in the future:

Father, thank You that I stand before You completely forgiven. My sins have been covered by the precious blood of Jesus, and I am now holy and blameless in Your sight.

Lord, I am calling on the name of the One who saved and forgave me of my sins. I am making a decision to forgive [insert name here] for [insert the offense the person committed]. In the name of Jesus, I completely forgive this person.

Father, thank You for giving me the power to forgive [insert name here]. I give You praise and honor for setting my heart free from the chain of unforgiveness. Jesus, please heal and restore my heart and fill me with Your love.

DAY 5: Going to the Cross

This week's lesson is designed to help us experience healing from our heart wounds; however, we may need to allow ourselves more than one week to work through these steps. We may also need to talk to and pray with someone as we work through these difficult issues.

The steps we have walked through will help us receive healing and freedom from past wounds, but they will also serve as a guide to help us know how to respond to future wounds.

➤ For review, what is the first step in healing a wounded heart?

Accepting healing

➤ What is the second step in healing a wounded heart?

Trusting God

➤ The third step in healing a wounded heart is to surrender our wound to Christ. In your own words, what does that mean?

Admitting them to God and to ourselves, praying (asking) for healing) Let God take care of it.

Like trusting God, surrendering a wound to Christ is a choice we make. We can choose to hold on to the wound, along with the pain and bondage that accompany it, or we can choose to give the wound to Christ.

➤ What benefits do we receive if we choose to hold on to a wound?

bondage, pain, fear, worry, doubt

➤ What benefits do we receive if we surrender a wound to Christ?

freedom complete, peace, joy

➤ Prayerfully consider the words of God in Psalm 62:8. What do you think it means to trust in God at all times?

We can trust God w/every thing that come into our life, to help us handle & get through

What do you think it means to pour out your heart to God?

He is my best friend, I can tell Him everything (He knows anyway) I can trust Him.

Why do you think God tells us He is our refuge when we trust Him and pour our hearts out to Him?

He hides us from harm, heart and danger. He protects us from the enemy.

➳ Imagine that your heart is a cup and that you are turning that cup upside down before Christ. What emotions would you like to keep from spilling out before Christ?

None!

The emotions that you listed are the precise emotions that need to be poured out before Christ. Those are the emotions that Christ wants to take from you. Anger, insecurity, fear and pride may be some of the emotions that you have not given to God. God doesn't want you holding on to those emotions. He wants you to pour your heart out to Him.

➳ Read Isaiah 61:3,7. These verses recount the beautiful exchanges that have taken place because of Christ's work on the cross. List these exchanges in the space provided.

③ *beauty / Ashes*
   gladness / morning
   praise / despair

② *double portion / shame*
   inheritance / disgrace
   Joy

For the remainder of today's lesson, we are going to take a trip to the Cross. Please go to your altar with a pen and your journal or a piece of paper.

Close your eyes and imagine that you are sitting at the foot of the cross. Thank Jesus for dying for you and for giving you a new life. Thank Him for wanting to heal you and free you. Tell Jesus that you want Him to heal your heart. Tell Jesus how the wounds have made you feel; do not hold back any thoughts or feelings. Pour your heart out to God.

Now imagine that you are taking your wounds into your hands and laying them at Jesus' feet. Surrender the wounds and all the painful emotions to Him. This is the time for exchange. Jesus has taken your wounds in exchange for your healing and freedom.

Ask Jesus to heal your heart, to restore all that the wounds have taken from your heart and to fill your heart with His love and grace. Spend time thanking and praising Jesus for the work He has done in your life today.

> **Note:** If this step is difficult for you, write a letter to Jesus in your journal. Tell Him about the wound you bear, how it makes you feel and how it has affected your life.

Be sensitive to what God wants to do in your life. You may have an especially deep wound that needs several trips to the Cross. God knows the best time for you to work through each wound. Remember the words of Proverbs 3:5-6; the Lord promises to direct us as we trust Him with all our hearts.

 Father God, You declare that I am blessed because I do not walk in the counsel of the wicked. My delight is in Your Word and I meditate on it both day and night. I am like a tree planted by a stream of water that yields its fruit in season and whose leaf does not wither. Thank You for causing me to prosper [see Psalm 1:1-3].

DAY 6: *Reflections*

This week we have identified and taken steps toward healing wounds in our hearts. This path to healing may have produced feelings of vulnerability. Allowing God to reveal wounds that need His healing can initially stir up emotions such as fear, anxiety, doubt and confusion. Often the first thing we do when faced with unpleasant emotions is seek comfort in food. It is so important to realize that we have a choice when it comes to dealing with unpleasant emotions. We can turn to food or we can turn to God.

Our memory verse is a promise from God that we can cling to when our hearts feel vulnerable or troubled. God tells us that He is with us. We may feel alone, but the truth is that we are never alone. The Lord is with us and He is mighty. The Lord rescues our hearts from the most furious storms.

Not only does the Lord save us, but He also delights in us. When we feel alone or discouraged, we need to remind ourselves that God sees us as His beautiful masterpieces. The Lord will quiet the storm in our hearts when we embrace His love. Hope and peace will replace despair and worry when we believe that God celebrates over us with love songs from His heart. Choose to believe God's Word instead of your negative thoughts and feelings.

Dear Father, though the path may be difficult at times, I want nothing more that to continue on this journey to complete freedom. When Satan attacks me, draw me close to You and quiet my heart with Your love.

Thank You, Lord, for continuing the work You have begun in my life.

DAY 7: *Reflections*

Today you have a special assignment: Write a love letter to Jesus. God has written many love letters to you, kept bound and preserved in the pages of the Bible, and today it is His turn to get one from you. Don't skip this assignment—you will be blessed as you express your love to your Savior. You may use the space provided or your journal.

Dear Jesus,

_____

_____

_____

_____

_____

_____

_____

_____

Love,

Precious Lord, You are the lover of my soul. Your love for me is incomprehensible, and it fills my heart with quiet longing for You.

Jesus, may You take great delight in my love offering to You.

NAME	REQUEST	RESULTS
Debbie		
Becky H.	traveling	
Teresa's parent	health	
Jo Melissa	Caley	
Lisa	Debbie's sister	
Thompson's	Anthony 4/4 bone marrow tico	
Charlee Dobey	Burg - mon	
John McDaniel		

BREAK DOWN STRONGHOLDS

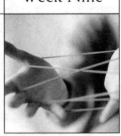

MEMORY VERSE

*We demolish arguments and every pretension that sets
itself up against the knowledge of God, and we take
captive every thought to make it obedient to Christ.*

2 Corinthians 10:5

The Lord our God demonstrated His passion for our freedom through the
death and resurrection of His beloved Son, Jesus Christ. The death and
resurrection of Christ set us completely free from the power of sin and
death. Because of the Cross we are now new creations in Christ. As we
continue our study of strongholds this week, let's keep an attitude of
praise and thanksgiving for the gift and power of the Cross.

DAY 1: *Understanding Satan's Plan*

Recall from week six that though the term "stronghold" is sometimes
used to describe a fortress of safety from the enemy, 2 Corinthians 10:4
is referring to a stronghold built by our enemy to keep us imprisoned
and in bondage.

➼ If a stronghold can be built as protection from the enemy, and we
know that Satan "masquerades as an angel of light" (2 Corinthians
11:14), how do you think Satan wants us to view strongholds in our
lives? *maybe as prisons, something
to escape from.*

➼ Why do you think Satan wants us to believe that way?

*He wants us to have nothing
from God — no protection, no trust,
no dependance*

⨠ What is the truth about strongholds in our lives?

They can be a fortress if built by God or a prison if satan is allowed to build one in your life

⨠ How do you think strongholds affect our ability to live as new creations in Christ?

If we build our stronghold on the Word of God we have all the protection, peace, etc as we grow in Christ.

Read Genesis 3:1-8 to review how the enemy works in our lives. We have already identified the tools Satan used to deceive Eve into thinking that she was disobeying God to get life, when she was really getting death.

⨠ Read James 1:13-15. List the steps the enemy uses to entice us to death.

Temptation ② ⟵⟶ desire ① → sin → death

What do you think the word "death" means in these verses?

Seperation from God

⨠ Review John 10:10. What is Satan's plan for our lives?

To steal, kill & destroy

What does this Scripture teach us about how Satan attempts to fulfill his plan for our lives?

He is deceptive, little steps at a time until he has built His stronghold in our lives

It is so important to recognize how Satan works in our lives. We don't just wake up one day completely imprisoned by a stronghold. Satan works methodically and cunningly in our lives. Second Corinthians 2:11 states, "We are not unaware of his schemes." The word "scheme" means "a crafty or secret plan or program of action."[1] God knows Satan's plan of action, and He wants us to be aware of it too.

➤ Why do you think it is important for us to be aware of Satan's plan of action? *As in any battle, it is important to plan a defence. Being aware, HE is OUT THERE, trying to defeat God's PLAN for your life.*

➤ Based on what you have studied today, describe Satan's method for building a stronghold in your life.

Sneaking in, little by little, one brick @ a time until we are imprisoned.

➤ Read 2 Corinthians 10:4. For review, what are the weapons with which we fight to gain victory in our lives?

divine power

What do these weapons attack?

strongholds

Father, I praise Your holy name. Thank You that all my sins are forgiven and that You heal all my diseases. You have redeemed my life from the pit, and I am crowned with Your love and compassion [see Psalm 103:1-4].

My God, thank You for revealing Satan's schemes for my destruction. Equip me to withstand the enemy's attacks and to resist his attempts to build strongholds in my life.

DAY 2: *Understanding Generational Sin*

Yesterday we learned that Satan has a plan of action for building strongholds in our lives. He wants to use those strongholds to lead us away from God and into bondage.

We do not all share the same struggles in life. Not everyone struggles with food addictions. Some people struggle with pride, low self-esteem, jealousy, chemical addictions or materialism. Not everyone is tempted by the same fruit. Satan knows our individual weaknesses and what fruit to dangle in front of us.

➤ With what thoughts, attitudes and actions does Satan tempt you?

All kinds. materialism, vengence being judgmental

Our enemy keeps a record of our failures in life. He also keeps a record of the failures of our parents and grandparents. Part of Satan's method for building strongholds in our lives is taking advantage of opportunities he has been given through our parents' and grandparents' sin; i.e., generational sin.

➤ Please read Exodus 34:6-7. According to these verses, how can the unconfessed sins of our parents and grandparents affect us today?

Can you get above your raisins'? How we are taught growing up we carry w/us always.

➤ According to Proverbs 20:7, what does God promise the righteous?

A blameless life

What do you think God means by a "blameless life"?

A person is saved by the blood of Christ, he claims that blood for forgiveness of confessed sin

It is impossible for us to live lives free of sin. We are righteous, holy and blameless before God only because the blood of Jesus covers us.

➺ Look back at Exodus 34:6-7. What does God tell us that He is willing to forgive?

Wickedness, rebellion and sin.

➺ Read 1 John 1:9. How do we receive forgiveness for the sins that we commit? *Confession*

God is full of compassion and mercy, but He will not ignore sin. Our children will experience the consequences of sin that we attempt to hide from God, the same way we experience the consequences of the sin our parents and grandparents attempted to hide from God.

➺ Do you recognize any struggles in your life that your parents and/or grandparents also struggled with? Explain.

Both my grandparents + my parents were coniving. I find myself thinking that way sometimes.

Generational alcoholism is generally accepted by our culture as hereditary. A quick temper is considered to be a personality trait passed down from a family member, but the Lord sees both alcoholism and a quick temper as sins.

➺ How do you think Satan uses generational sin in his scheming?

Affects your thinking. My parents did it and lived through it. I can get by w/this

Jesus bore all sin on the cross. He took upon Himself generational sins, sins we commit today and sins we will commit tomorrow. Jesus' blood covers all of them.

If you question whether you are suffering from generational sin, ask God to reveal it. We have learned that God exposes hidden things. Remember, the Lord is passionate about your freedom. If you are in bondage because of generational sin, God wants to expose it to you.

Spend some time in prayer. You can use the following prayer or your own words. Remember to pray aloud.

My Father, Lord and Savior, I humble myself before You. Thank You for rescuing me and giving me a new life. Lord, I want to be free from any generational sin that Satan would wish to use against me. Please reveal to me any generational sin that is affecting my life today. In the powerful name of Jesus, Amen.

Write down anything that God reveals to you, and then pray the following prayer aloud for each generational sin God revealed.

Father, thank You for exposing this sin in my life. Lord, I confess [insert the sin] and ask that You forgive me and my family for this sin. I demand in the name of Jesus that all work of the enemy because of this sin be removed from my life and from the lives of my family. Father, I ask You to completely break the curses of this generational sin, in the name of Jesus.

Thank You, Lord, that I am completely free from this generational sin. All punishment has been cancelled. The work of the enemy has been destroyed and I am free. Lord, I ask You to fill my heart with Your Holy Spirit and consume my mind with Your truth. In Jesus' name, amen.

Generational sin certainly gives Satan an opportunity to build a stronghold in our lives. He would like us to accept struggles and unpleasant personality traits as part of life or deny them altogether. However, God wants us to view sin as the destructive and ugly thing it is. When we see sin as sin, we step out of denial. The next step we take must be toward the Cross. At the Cross we find forgiveness, healing and victory.

 Father God, thank You that I have been given everything I need because You have given me the fullness of Christ, who is the head over every power and authority [see Colossians 2:10].

DAY 3: Building Strongholds

We learned yesterday that Satan tries to use generational sin to create strongholds in our lives. Today we will discover how we put ourselves in bondage by allowing strongholds to develop in our lives.

The following is a list of some common strongholds in people's lives:

- Alcohol
- Anger
- Depression
- Drugs
- Fear
- Food
- Guilt
- Idolatry

- Legalism
- Overspending
- People-pleasing
- Pride
- Selfish ambition
- Sexual addictions
- Unforgiveness

gambling

> What other strongholds come to your mind?

Busyness, stress, apathy

> Look again at James 1:13-15, paying close attention to verse 14. When are we tempted?

When we pay attention to our own evil desire

What is the condition of our hearts before we are tempted?

Thinking about our desires

Where do our "evil desire[s]" come from?

The desire within us and satan feed it.

> Based on what we have already learned from Psalm 37:4 about our desires (see week two, Day 4), what is one of the ways that we can protect our hearts from "evil desire[s]"?

Delight in the Lord always

➡ Look back at James 1:14. What do you think we are "dragged away" from?

from delighting in the Lord.

What occurs when we are dragged away?

sin & death (spiritual)

Recall how Satan worked in Eve's life. He made the apple enticing, or attractive, to her, and then he dragged her away from God's truth by causing her to doubt and become confused.

➡ Reread James 1:15. What do you think it means for desire to conceive?

make it happen

The word "conceived" in this verse is derived from a Greek word that can mean "to become pregnant."[2] At this point, the evil desire has not produced sin. The evil desire has developed into an evil seed within our hearts. There is still time to remove the seed in our lives before the seed becomes sin.

➡ How do you think we can remove the seed from our hearts before the seed, or desire, gives birth to sin?

Ask God to help us not give in to the desire.

➡ Look back at James 1:15. What do you think it means for sin to become "full-grown"?

You are in satans stronghold. You have made your desire happen.

What is the result of sin that has reached full growth? *death*

James 1:13-15 reveals how a stronghold is built. Let's review these steps together:

1. We entertain evil desires.
2. We are dragged away from following God and His Word.

3. We are enticed, or tempted, by the enemy.

4. We allow the desire to conceive.

5. We sin.

6. Our sin becomes full grown.

7. Death—a stronghold takes root in our life.

➤ According to 1 Corinthians 10:13, what does God promise us?

He will provide a way of escape.

We need to know some important truths about the enemy's strongholds. First, we have plenty of opportunities to escape before sin reaches full growth and results in a stronghold in our lives. Sin has to be allowed in our lives for an extended period of time to reach its full growth.

➤ How might generational sin affect the speed at which a sin reaches full growth? Explain.

If you have been taught you can have & deserve to have, you might seize this sin more quickly.

We also need to know this truth: We can safeguard ourselves from the development of a stronghold.

➤ Look back at the steps of building a stronghold. What could we do after step 5 that would hinder the growth process?

I John 1:9

➤ Look at the first two steps in building a stronghold. How can we entirely avoid the work of the enemy in our lives?

Spend much time w/the LORD Quote memory verses.

Desiring to be, and choosing to live as, new creations in Christ is a daily choice and is the only way to safeguard our lives from strongholds.

 Lord, You are my portion and I promise to obey Your words. I have sought Your face with all my heart; thank You for being gracious to me according to Your promises. Since I have considered the error in my ways and have turned my steps to Your statutes, I will not delay to obey Your commands [see Psalm 119:57-60].

DAY 4: *Revealing Strongholds*

We have learned through studying Scripture that God will expose and reveal to us the deep and hidden things in our hearts. When we invite God to examine our thoughts, beliefs and lives, He is faithful to show us what we need to be healed and freed from. God reveals these things to us because He passionately wants us to experience His healing and freedom.

Revealing the strongholds that oppress us is the next step in our freedom. Today we will ask God to reveal any strongholds in our lives. Tomorrow we will learn how to remove those strongholds.

Ask God to reveal any strongholds in your life. Use the following prayer or your own words. Remember to pray out loud.

Father, thank You for being so passionate about my healing and freedom, and for sending Jesus to give me eternal life in heaven and abundant life on Earth. I desire to walk in complete freedom from any strongholds that are in my life. Father, I ask You to reveal any strongholds that are keeping me from that freedom. Thank You for speaking clearly and specifically to my heart. In the name of Jesus, amen.

➤ List any strongholds that God revealed to you during your time of prayer.

busyness

When we cultivate a stronghold, we also simultaneously develop a conscious or unconscious belief system about it. The next step to freedom from a stronghold is to identify the false belief system that helped build the stronghold. For example, if food addiction is a stronghold in your life, ask God to identify what beliefs were involved in developing that stronghold.

Using the following prayer or your own words, ask God to reveal any lies that you believe about the strongholds you listed. As you pray aloud, use the space provided following the prayer to write any lies that God reveals to you.

Father, I want to walk in Your truth. I confess that [insert stronghold] has competed with You for first place in my life. I choose to serve You and have no other gods before You. I want to be free from any form of idolatry in my life. Lord, I ask You to reveal any lies that I have believed about [insert stronghold] and what it can do for me and my life. I ask this in the name of Jesus, amen.

It's okay, you have to take care of things. The bed has to be changed, the house spotless. You have to cook.

Once the lies have been revealed, we know the next step: Renounce the lies and seek forgiveness. Pray the following prayer aloud:

Father, thank You for revealing to me the lies that I believe about [insert stronghold]. I renounce the lie that [insert the lie]. I ask You to forgive me for believing and serving this lie. I refuse to believe this lie any longer, and now I choose to walk in Your truth. In Jesus' name, amen.

➤ How might the strongholds in your life affect your goals in First Place?

*No time for exercise.
No time to eat right.
No time to pray effectually
etc.*

> ➤ How does worshiping food or any other stronghold affect your ability
> to live as a new creation?

Thou shalt have no other gods before me.

> ➤ Why do you think the enemy would use something like food to create
> a stronghold in your life?

Anything to build his stronghold.

Tomorrow we will further discuss the process of removing strongholds. But before we end today's lesson, spend a few moments in prayer thanking God for all the work He has been accomplishing in your life. Write your prayer in the space provided or in your journal.

DAY 5: *Removing Strongholds*

We have learned that a stronghold is an area of our life that the enemy uses to keep us in bondage. We know that strongholds are developed over time and that generational sin can accelerate the building process. Yesterday we learned how strongholds have developed in our lives and uncovered our false beliefs about them. Today we will learn how to remove those strongholds from our lives. Some of this lesson will be review, but the information is critical to this stage.

> ➤ Look again at 2 Corinthians 10:4. What kinds of weapons do we use
> to demolish strongholds? *divine weapons*

A stronghold is much like a building. Tools of deception lay the foundation; then sin, false beliefs and denial build the tower that holds us captive.

➤ What does God tell us our weapons will do to strongholds (v. 4)?

demolish them

The power of the Holy Spirit, prayer and God's Word are the weapons that we use to demolish strongholds. God can allow those weapons to completely demolish a stronghold with one attack. However, God may desire that we use His weapons to dismantle a stronghold piece by piece over time.

➤ Why do you think God sometimes desires us to dismantle a stronghold piece by piece?

God knows us better than anyone. He knows what works

What do you think God may want to accomplish in our lives through that process?

His will, trust Him + obey

➤ Why do you think God sometimes chooses immediate deliverance from a stronghold in our life?

Same thing. He knows our need.

God may choose immediate deliverance from a stronghold or He may choose to walk us through the steps of deliverance over time. God knows which form of deliverance will accomplish the work He wants to do in each of our lives.

➤ What are we promised in Psalm 72:12?

deliverence

If God has revealed that food addiction is a stronghold in your life, the following prayer will help you break down that stronghold; you may also modify this prayer to fit other strongholds. You may need to say this prayer daily until you feel a release in your life, and especially when you feel weak or tempted. The prayer includes Scriptures that you can use daily to renew your mind. You may want to go to your altar to pray.

 Father, Your Word promises that when I commit whatever I do to You, my plans will succeed [see Proverbs 16:3]. Lord, I commit to serve You and love You with all my heart. I refuse to be mastered by food. I choose to throw off everything that hinders me, including this sin that so easily entangles me, and to patiently run the race before me. I am fixing my eyes on Jesus, the author and finisher of my faith [see Hebrews 12:1-2].

I have been declared free, and I will not use my freedom to indulge my sinful nature [see Galatians 5:13]. I refuse to deceive myself by merely listening to Your Word; I commit to doing what Your Word says [see James 1:22]. I know that what You are commanding me to do today is not too difficult for me or beyond my reach [see Deuteronomy 30:11]. Thanks be to God! You give me victory through my Lord, Jesus Christ [see 1 Corinthians 15:57].

DAY 6: Reflections

We are one week away from the conclusion of this study. Let's reflect on what we have learned over the past nine weeks. Please take a few moments to prayerfully consider the following questions. You do not need to write responses. Simply ponder what the Lord has taught you through the study of His Word.

- What is a new creation in Christ?
- How do you desire to live as a new creation in Christ?
- What is the significance of choosing to live as a new creation in Christ?
- What are some obstacles to living as a new creation in Christ?
- How can you exercise your given authority?
- How is your life transformed so that you can live as a new creation in Christ?

- Describe the heart of God.
- How does God heal a wounded heart?
- How are strongholds broken down?

Father, thank You for working for my good and for Your purpose in all things because I love You [see Romans 8:28]. Thank You for the work You have done in my life.

DAY 7: *Reflections*

We know that we are transformed by the renewing of our minds (see Romans 12:2). The following is a list of "Truth Treasures." Spend a few moments reading these treasures aloud to yourself.

I am God's treasured possession (see Deuteronomy 7:6).

I am blessed and surrounded with God's favor (see Psalm 5:12).

I am the apple of God's eye (see Psalm 17:8).

I am fearfully and wonderfully made (see Psalm 139:14).

My name is engraved on the palm of God's hands (see Isaiah 49:16).

I have been clothed with Christ (see Galatians 3:27).

I am a saint (see Ephesians 1:1).

Thank God for His Word and receive His truth for you today. Look back on these verses when the enemy tries to deceive you with thoughts of self-doubt. Hide these words in your heart—they will keep you from sin and help you guard against strongholds (see Psalm 119:11).

Father God, Your Word is perfect and it revives my soul. Your commands give light to my eyes and bring joy to my heart. Help me to obey Your Word so that I may receive the great reward You reserve for the righteous [see Psalm 19:7-8,11].

Notes

1. *Merriam-Webster's Collegiate Dictionary*, 11th ed., s.v. "scheme."
2. James Strong, *The Strongest Strong's Exhaustive Concordance of the Bible* (Grand Rapids, MI: Zondervan Publishing House, 2001), Greek #4815.

GROUP PRAYER REQUESTS   TODAY'S DATE:_____

NAME	REQUEST	RESULTS
Holly		
Charlee		
Ann Steffy		
Janice's dad + mom (ears)		
Aleta - 5yr (Mary Sloanes)	Spinabifia	
Diane's family		
Mary's house		
Jay's neices -		

FULFILL HIS PURPOSES

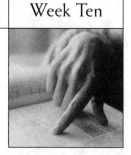

MEMORY VERSE
And we, who with unveiled faces all reflect the Lord's glory, are being transformed into his likeness with ever-increasing glory, which comes from the Lord, who is the Spirit.
2 Corinthians 3:18

God has given us a new identity through our relationship with Him, making us new creations in Christ. We have learned through God's Word that to live as new creations in Christ, we must allow Christ to live through us. Our lives become Christ's vessels when we empty ourselves and allow Christ to fill us, heal us and make us fit for His service.

God has several purposes for creating us with the ability to be vessels for Christ. We will look at some of those purposes this week.

DAY 1: *A Servant's Heart*

Today we will discover God's first purpose for making us new creations as we study an attribute of Christ that marked His entire life on Earth.

➤ Read 2 Corinthians 1:3-4. What is one of the reasons that God comforts us?

So that we can comfort others

In what way are we to comfort others?

*Empathy
Compassion
Mercy*

*Prayer
scriptures - favorite
verses*

❧ Can you think of someone whom you have been able to comfort because of the compassion and comfort that God showed you during a troubling time? Explain.

Last week - Joy
Mandy - lost baby

❧ Read Philippians 2:1-4. What qualities do we receive when we are united with Christ (v. 1)?

encouragement
comfort from His love
fellowship with the Spirit
tenderness & compassion

What are we encouraged to do with these gifts (v. 2)?

Be like-minded - show these
gifts to others

Having received these gifts, what are we warned to avoid (v. 3)? Why do you think we are warned to avoid these things?

selfish ambition
vain conceit = pride
Humanity makes us vol

❧ How can the instructions found in verse 4 safeguard us from becoming prideful and having selfish ambition?

look for at the needs in others

❧ What do you think it means to consider others better than yourself (v. 3)?

humility

❧ Read Philippians 2:5-8. We are told in verse 5 that our attitudes toward others should be like Christ's. According to this passage, what example did Christ give us?

That of a servant
Humility - Obedience

➤ Read Philippians 2:9-11. How did God bless His Son's humble obedience to death?

He exalted Him

➤ Read the following verses. In the space provided, note what each passage says about humility.

Psalm 25:9   *He guides and teaches*

Psalm 149:4   *He crowns the humble w/ salvation*

James 4:10   *Humble yourself and He will lift you up*

1 Peter 5:5-6   *God gives grace to the humble*

➤ How do you think humility affects our ability to serve others?

True humility = a servant's heart

God puts people in our lives for us to serve. However, we can't do it in our own strength—we are to serve them with the grace and love of Christ that flow through our lives. Walking in truth and freedom allows the love of Christ to permeate our lives, enabling us to pass that love to others.

Ask God to show you the people He has put in your life to serve. Close today's lesson in prayer. Thank God for trusting you to share His

love and grace with others and ask Him to help and strengthen you.
Write your prayer in the space provided or in your journal.

DAY 2: *A Fruitful Life*

Today we will discover another of the purposes God has for His new creations: to bear fruit in our lives that resembles Christ's.

➤ Read John 15:1-12. In this metaphor, who is the gardener and what are His responsibilities?

> My Heavenly Father - He prunes
> He ~~is~~ the lifeline
> provided

Who is the vine and what is His responsibility?

> ~~We are~~. We are to stay
> Jesus Christ

➤ Who are the branches? What must they do to bear fruit?

> We are. Remain in Him

What is the result of bearing fruit (v. 8)?

> showing we are disciples of Christ

➤ Why does Jesus want us to obey His commands (vv. 10-11)?

> so that His joy and our joy
> may be complete.

➤ In 1 John 5:3, how are God's commands described?

> Not burdensome

➤ Reread John 15:12-13. What particular fruit does Jesus want us to bear?

reproducing His love

➤ Read Mark 12:28-31. Why do you think this fruit is so important that Jesus deemed it the second greatest commandment?

In seeing His love in you, they see Him.

➤ Read 1 John 4:15-17. Explain how abiding in Christ will ensure that we can successfully bear the fruit of love.

His love flows through us.

Love → → → STAY ATTACHED
Vine
us

Some people are easy to love and to feel an affinity toward, while others seem impossible to love. However, God's supply of love is unlimited; and when we abide in Christ, we are enabled to love the unlovable.

➤ Look back at John 15:16-17. How does Jesus describe the fruit we must bear?

Fruit that remains

Why is it important to bear this kind of fruit (v. 16)?

God choose and appointed us to represent Him and share His love to a lost mankind. Other than

In your own words, describe what it means to bear this kind of fruit.

divine revelation there is no other way for lost MAN TO FIND CHRIST

➤ Look again at verse John 15:2. What do you suppose it means that the gardener, God, "prunes" the branches that bear fruit?

Some things in our life are not needed. They may not be sinful, but they may weigh us down so that our fruit bearing is hindered. God may need to take them out of our life. It may hurt, but we will bear more.

Why do you think He does this?

To make us more fruitful

>> Based on all you have learned through this study, how do we abide in Christ?

Inviting Him & desiring Him to work through us daily.
A servant's heart, a fruitful life

In closing today, ask God to examine the fruit that you bear in your life. Are you abiding in Christ and producing eternal fruit? Are you allowing the gardener to prune you—to remove what needs removing? Are you seeking to know and follow God's precepts? Is there someone in your life whom you need God's help to love? God wants you to grow and flourish so that others may come to know His great love.

Father God, thank You for showing me the best way to love. I want Your love to flow through me so that my love is patient and kind. Keep rudeness, anger and evil far from my heart. Your love always protects, trusts, hopes and perseveres. Teach me to love others the way that You love me [see 1 Corinthians 13:4-7].

DAY 3: A Living Testament

Let's look back at one of our memory verses, Ephesians 2:10. In this verse, Paul reminds us that as God's children we are His workmanship. Recall from week seven that the word "workmanship" is derived from the Greek word "poiema," from which we derive the English word "poem."

>> According to Ephesians 2:10, what is the purpose of our poet's poem?

good works

➤ Read 2 Corinthians 3:1-3. The apostle Paul was writing to the church
in Corinth. How did Paul describe the people to whom he ministered?

a letter from Christ

Where had this ministry taken place?

Tablets of the human heart

What did Paul use to minister to these people? *letters*

spirit of the living God

➤ Read 2 Corinthians 3:4-6. Describe Paul's attitude toward his ministry. *tiful*

(Beau-
verses

Confidence through Christ
competent because of God

The word "competent" means "having adequate ability or qualities."[1]
Paul is saying that he is equipped and capable as a minister of the new
covenant.

➤ Why do you think Paul was so sure of his ability to minister?

Because he was depending on
God. His confidence came because
of his trust

What can you learn from Paul's example that will help you minister to
people in your home and in your life?

Depend on God, pray a lot, ask for
His help and wisdom

➤ Name some of the people in your life to whom you minister.

Shut-ins, high maintence friends

In what ways do you minister to them?

Prayer, counseling, prepare food

➤ Read 1 Corinthians 15:58. How can knowing that your labor in the Lord is not in vain help you the next time you are discouraged and don't see immediate fruit from your labor?

This is Paul, speaking for God, in our corner, cheering for us.

One of the most powerful ways we can serve and minister to others is through prayer.

➤ Read James 5:16. How does God describe our prayers?

powerful and effective.

Go to your altar for the purpose of ministering to others through prayer. Ask God to show you whom He wants you to pray for today. Lift those loved ones up in prayer knowing that your prayers are powerful and effective. You can use the following prayer or your own words.

Father God, I lift up [insert person's name] to you. Thank You for putting [insert person's name] in my life. I pray that [insert person's name] will experience a greater revelation of Your love. Give [insert person's name] discernment to know what is best for [his or her] life. Keep [insert person's name] pure and blameless until the day of Christ's return and fill [insert person's name] with the fruit of righteousness that comes through Jesus Christ [see Philippians 1:9-11].

DAY 4: A Life of Blessings

God receives glory when He showers our lives with blessings—when He meets our needs, gives us strength and peace in the middle of a storm, fills our hearts with joy and hope in the midst of a trial, when He changes our hearts and transforms our lives. God desires to bless His new creations because it brings Him glory and because He loves us dearly.

➤ List the many blessings that God has given us as found in Ephesians 1:3-14. Use more paper if necessary.

Chosen *riches of His grace*
adopted *revelation - His will*
redeemed *promise of future*
forgiven

According to verse 4, how does God see us?

holy & blameless

➤ Review Ephesians 4:22-24. How does God describe His <u>new</u> creations?

righteous & holy

➤ According to 1 Peter 2:9, who does God say you are?

a chosen people, a royal priesthood, a holy nation, a people belonging to God.

➤ Read Romans 3:22-25. What does your new position in life cost you?

Nothing

What did your new position in life cost God?

His Son - all

➤ Based on all you have learned through this study, why do you think God paid the price to give you your new position?

He loves me and it gives Him glory

➤ What did God reveal about Himself through His own sacrifice?

His great love

What does that tell us about God's desire to bless us?

He desires to do so

➤ Read Deuteronomy 11:26-28. What must we do to receive God's blessings?

Be obedient to His commands

God's Word is a tremendous blessing in our lives. However, we don't receive that blessing unless we choose daily to read God's Word and believe what it tells us.

➤ How has studying God's Word helped you as a First Place member?

It shows me that He will help me, if I ask. I am a new creation in Him, and I can do all things

➤ How has studying God's Word helped you to see your life differently?

It makes me realize how unworthy I am, but God loves me and wants me to be happy & succeed.

➤ How has studying God's Word helped you to see others differently?

God loves and forgives. I should, too

➤ How has studying God's Word helped you to better understand the greatest of all blessings: God's love and the love of His beloved Son?

How can you answer that in this small space, even if I could adequately put it into words

How has this revelation of God's love and the love of Christ affected you?

I stand in awe of Him. I want to worship and serve Him. I want to represent Him to others my great and mighty God love us all

God deeply desires to bless you. He couldn't possibly have given you a greater blessing than the life of His dearly loved Son. If you are still having difficulty receiving the blessing of God's great love for you, please pray this prayer daily until you can fully embrace the truth of His amazing love for you.

Father, I want to know Your great love for me. You know my heart and You know the walls that are separating me from receiving the fullness of Your love. I ask You to remove those walls and to fill my heart with Your love.

God, reveal Your heart to me in a greater way each day. Create in me a passion to love You with everything in me.

DAY 5: *A Firm Stand*

For our final lesson we will study the importance of standing firm in the position that we have been given as new creations in Christ.

➤ Based on 2 Corinthians 5:17 and all you have learned through God's Word, describe who you are as a new creation in Christ.

Heir & joint-heir w/ Jesus
A chosen vessel, forgiven, redeemed & adopted

➤ Read Galatians 5:1. What are we instructed to do and not to do?

Stand firm and do not let yourselves be burdened by the yoke of slavery

➤ List some of the things that Christ has set you free from.

Rom. 6:18,22 - free from sin
John 8:32 - The TRUTH shall set you free from strongholds

For what purpose has Christ set you free?

To honor & glorify Him

We have studied in detail the effects strongholds have on our lives. Strongholds keep us in bondage. Praise God, Jesus came to set us free and break the "yoke of slavery."

> According to Galatians 5:1, how do we remain free?

Stand firm

The enemy is waiting for the ideal time to lay a familiar trap for a child of God who has been set free.

> Read 1 Peter 5:8-9. How is Satan described (v. 8)?

Roaring lion

What instructions does God give us regarding how to withstand our enemy's attacks?

Be self-controlled + alert

> What have you learned about your thought life, prayer and God's Word that will help you follow those instructions?

Be deligent to guard your thoughts, pray and read +meditate on the Word

Recall that the enemy has tools, or weapons, that he uses against us. Deception is Satan's favorite weapon. He does all he can to get us to believe his lies. God tells us to resist and refuse those lies. Do not believe them! Cast them away and use God's Word to completely destroy their power and renew your mind.

First Peter 5:9 also tells us that our "brothers [and sisters] throughout the world are undergoing the same kind of sufferings."

> How can knowing this truth comfort you when you are under attack?

Elijah Thinking about them and what they are going thru make you know you're not the only one.

> Read 1 Peter 5:10. What does God promise to do for us?

He will restore us. He will make us strong, firm + steadfast.

We are new creations in Christ. We have been given victory over sin and death. We are declared free by the blood of Jesus. We have been given the power and authority through the Holy Spirit, prayer and God's Word to walk in complete healing and freedom. And God receives great joy when His new creations walk in His truth.

Father God, thank You that I am a new creation in Christ [see 2 Corinthians 5:17], that I have been given victory over sin and death [see Romans 6:23], that I am declared free by the blood of Jesus and that I have been given the power and authority through the Holy Spirit, prayer and God's Word to walk in complete healing and freedom.

I pray, Lord, that You would receive glory and be filled with joy as I walk in Your truth.

DAY 6: *Reflections*

Jesus came to set God's people free. There is not a sin, a stronghold, a wound, a lie, an obstacle or an enemy that has the power to keep us enslaved or in bondage. God's Word tells us that we are "transformed into his likeness with ever-increasing glory, which comes from the Lord, who is the Spirit" (2 Corinthians 3:18). God wants to reveal His glory to us at an ever-increasing level in our lives. God passionately wants our lives to be transformed into a greater likeness of His Son.

Our enemy does not want us to pursue more and more of Christ. Being content or complacent in our walk with Christ is a trick of the devil. Complacency keeps us from seeking the heart of God with passion, especially when the demands of life compete for our time. Remember, our enemy has tools to distract us from God. There are obstacles in our daily lives that a complacent heart will not have the strength to overcome.

When we seek Christ through prayer and God's Word and yield to the work of the Holy Spirit, God's glory will be revealed in our lives. Our lives will become more of a reflection of Christ as we are transformed into His likeness. The world will see the glory of God revealed in our lives. Hallelujah!

Father, thank You for setting me free. I know the road ahead may be difficult because Satan would like nothing more than to see me become complacent and enslaved once again. Don't let him succeed.

God, continue to transform me into the likeness of Your Son. Give me the strength to resist the devil's attempts to enslave me.

DAY 7: *Reflections*

As we conclude this study, take some time to pray and ask God to reveal the changes He has made in your life. List those positive changes in the space provided or in your journal.

Regular Bible Study
Praying more effectively because of the knowledge of His Word

Now ask God to show you the areas of your life in which He would still like to help you make changes. List those areas in the space provided or in your journal.

More compassion

We need to apply the principles of this study daily to live as new creations in Christ. We must desire and choose to live in the freedom God has given us by walking in His truth, by refusing to bow down to the lies of the enemy, by allowing Christ to restore our wounded hearts and by recognizing obstacles in our lives and exercising our given authority to remove them.

As new creations in Christ we have much to celebrate! We have been given freedom, a new identity and eternal life. Close your study with a trip to your altar. Spend time praising and thanking God for all He has done in your life through Christ over the past 10 weeks.

Father God, Your love for me is astounding. I would still be in darkness and bondage were it not for Your mercy. Continue to guide me daily into Your truth.

May You receive all the glory and praise for the work You have done—and will continue to do—in my life.

Note
1. *Merriam-Webster's Collegiate Dictionary*, 11th ed., s.v. "competent."

II Cor 12:9

Group Prayer Requests   Today's Date:_____

Name	Request	Results
Jimmy Montrose	Sarah's dad	
Anthony		
Adams, Lila family		
Brenda Frazier	Cheryl's patient	
Tammy Copley	Cheryl patient	
Leah's mom & Dad		
Teresa's parents		
Janice		
new Class		
Ruth Hale		

LEARNING TO MANAGE PAST FAILURE AND SUCCESS

Forgetting what is behind and straining toward what
is ahead, I press on toward the goal to win the prize for
which God has called me heavenward in Christ Jesus.
Philippians 3:13-14

Becoming new creations in Christ means that we need to put our pasts in proper perspective. Past failures have the power to paralyze us if we let them. Have you ever found yourself thinking, *I have failed so many times; I just don't have the courage to try again?* The fear of failure based on past experiences can keep us from success in the future.

Not only can past failure affect our progress, but so also can past successes. Have you ever found yourself thinking, *I lost weight before, but I know I can't be that successful again; I'm older now.* Past successes can place limitations on what God wants to do in our lives. We must adopt the apostle Paul's perspective on the past as he shared in Philippians 3:13-14: "Brothers [and sisters], I do not consider myself yet to have taken hold of it. But one thing I do: Forgetting what is behind and straining toward what is ahead, I press on toward the goal to win the prize for which God has called me heavenward in Christ Jesus."

Paul outlines three actions for us to emulate: forget what is behind, strain toward what is ahead and press on toward the prize.

FORGET WHAT IS BEHIND

What in Paul's life did he need to forget? Perhaps his successes, education or religious standing. Of course, even Paul had failures that could weigh him down if he were to dwell on them, such as his intense persecution of the Christians before he was saved.

≫ Identify at least one recent failure that has the potential to weigh you down. Does this failure cause you to doubt the transforming power of God in your life?

I lose, I gain back. Am I not trusting God or praying enough? I thank God I am healthy!

➤ We know that God has a purpose for everything. Can you think of a way in which God might use this failure to accomplish His plan in your life? Explain.

So that I can relate to others? Thorn in the flesh? (not possible, this is my own fault

Forgetting what is behind does not mean having spiritual amnesia, but it does mean that we will not allow the past to have power over us today.

STRAIN TOWARD WHAT IS AHEAD

Of what could Paul have been thinking when he said, "straining toward what is ahead"? Perhaps he was remembering the words of Jeremiah 29:11: "'For I know the plans I have for you,' declares the LORD, 'plans to prosper you and not to harm you, plans to give you hope and a future.'"

Perhaps Paul had called to mind the words of Isaiah 43:18-19: "Forget the former things; do not dwell on the past. See, I am doing a new thing! Now it springs up; do you not perceive it? I am making a way in the desert and streams in the wasteland." Do you believe these words of our great God and Savior?

Straining toward what is ahead means striving toward our bright new future! God is making a way in the desert for us to be successful.

➤ Identify one new thing that you have perceived God is doing in your life to turn your desert into an oasis.

Listening / absorbing. Because we know, we heard this before, we don't always listen to God or the preacher. You know what I mean. We listen, but we don't absorb.

PRESS ON TOWARD THE PRIZE

Pressing on means that we don't give up, even when it's hard. Deuteronomy 20:4 says, "For the LORD your God is the one who goes with you to fight for you against your enemies to give you victory." There are days when you will actually feel God pushing you with His strong right arm, helping you to press on.

➤ Identify at least one thing in your life that discourages you from pressing on.

weigh-in, failure

Now spend some time in prayer, asking God to push you past that discouragement and to help you keep pressing on, even in your weakest moments.

A NEW WAY OF THINKING

We must remember that we don't stand in victory because
of our faith, we stand in victory because of our God.
Beth Moore, *A Heart Like His*

Do you know that you can't think a positive thought and a negative thought at the same time? *Amazing*

How we think is central to the way we view ourselves. Becoming a new creation in Christ means transforming a depraved mind into one that is controlled by the Holy Spirit. Paul referred to this in Romans 8:6: "The mind of sinful man is death, but the mind controlled by the Spirit is life and peace." We can either choose to let the world and its circumstances rule our thoughts or to let God rule them.

The Bible provides a way to transform our way of thinking, but it requires some effort on our part.

STEP 1: REARRANGE YOUR THINKING

Words like "always" and "never" can be indicators of what psychologists call "imperative thinking"—a way of thinking that sets us up for failure. Perhaps a better name would be "stinking thinking." Read the thoughts below. Have you ever found yourself thinking any of the following statements?

It's no use; I am a failure.

Why should I even try again? I know I will never be able to finish the program.

There may be hope for others, but not for me.

My boss is right—I am just lazy!

See, I blew it again. I am such a loser!

Challenge these negative thoughts by focusing your thoughts on better things. Philippians 4:8 tells us, "Whatever is true, whatever is noble, whatever is right, whatever is pure, whatever is lovely, whatever is admirable—if anything is excellent or praiseworthy—think about such things."

There is a difference between positive thinking and positive faith. Ephesians 3:20 tells us that God is able to do much more than we can imagine, but we can't change by our good intentions alone; we are only transformed when we trust in the power of God within us—His Holy Spirit—and then take steps to walk in God's freedom.

STEP 2: GET RID OF FAULTY ASSUMPTIONS

The following statements are common assumptions people hold. Place a check mark by ones you think apply to you.

- ☐ *Everything I do should please others.*

- ☐ *If people around me are unhappy, it's probably my fault.*

- ☐ *God expects me to finish everything well without making any mistakes.*

- ☐ *I should not need others' help to succeed.*

- ☐ *What has happened to me in the past has determined my path for life and there's nothing I can do about it.*

- ☑ *If people could see the real me, they probably would not like me.*

The more thoughts you checked above, the more you will be hindered in your growth as a new creation. You need to replace those ungodly assumptions with godly truth so that you can continue to grow in Christ.

STEP 3: REPLACE LIES WITH TRUTH

Look at the following chart. In the left-hand column are common lies people believe. In the right-hand column are truths that replace those lies.

Lies	Truths
It is too hard for me to commit to anything. I am too busy and I don't have time.	If I commit my way to the Lord and trust in Him, He will give me the time. God is committed to those who are committed to Him.
I am not good at making wise decisions.	If I trust in the Lord with all my heart and acknowledge Him in all my ways, He will give me the direction and wisdom I need (see Proverbs 3:5-6).
I can't understand God.	I have been given the mind of Christ (see 1 Corinthians 2:16). I can better understand God with the help of the Holy Spirit and the Bible.

Are you still clinging to lies that need to be replaced with God's truth? Ask God to lead you in His truth to find a replacement for every lie you have believed.

DEVELOPING A HEALTHY SELF-IMAGE

Do you not know that your body is a temple of the Holy Spirit,
who is in you, whom you have received from God?
1 Corinthians 6:19

A healthy self-image is an important part of being a new creation in
Christ. Let's explore some steps that will help you realize who you truly
are in Christ.

STEP 1: REALIZE AND APPRECIATE YOUR UNIQUENESS

It's a proven fact: There is no one else exactly like you! You are uniquely
created to be one of a kind. Nothing about you is a mistake. Read the
psalmist's words regarding your individuality:

> For you created my inmost being; you knit me together in moth-
> er's womb. I praise you because I am fearfully and wonderfully
> made; your works are wonderful, I know that full well. My frame
> was not hidden from you when I was made in the secret place.
> When I was woven together in the depths of the earth, your eyes
> saw my unformed body. All the days ordained for me were written
> in your book before one of them came to be (Psalm 139:13-16).

➤ Identify something unique about yourself that sets you apart from others and that you could offer to God for His service.

Sacrificial service

Spend a few moments in prayer thanking God for your unique design
and for His intimate involvement in creating you.

STEP 2: THINK ABOUT WHAT IS TRUE

Another area in which people have many faulty assumptions is their appearance. In Wellness Worksheet Two we discussed replacing lies with truth. This exercise is similar. Take a look at the following faulty assumptions and truths to ponder:

> **Faulty Assumption**—Looks are central to who I am.
>
> **Truth to Ponder**—Consider wonderful people such as Corrie ten Boom, Billy Graham and Mother Teresa. Their looks are not the first thing you think of.
>
> **Faulty Assumption**—The first things people notice about my appearance are my imperfections.
>
> **Truth to Ponder**—Most people notice your best feature first. Remember, most people look better than they think they do!
>
> **Faulty Assumption**—Appearance always reflects the inner person.
>
> **Truth to Ponder**—Consider Christ. Scripture tells us there was nothing lovely about His appearance that would draw us to Him (see Isaiah 53:2).

Now it's your turn to apply what you've learned over the course of this study. The next two "Truth to Ponder" sections have been left blank for you to complete.

> **Faulty Assumption**—My appearance is responsible for much of what has happened to me.
>
> **Truth to Ponder**—
>
> **Faulty Assumption**—The only way I can ever be happy is to change the way I look.
>
> **Truth to Ponder**—

STEP 3: SEE YOUR BODY AS A GIFT

Let's do a little experiment. Close your eyes and picture yourself. Now suppose you were given the opportunity to ask God to change one thing about your body—what would you ask Him to change?

Now identify at least one thing about your physical body you really like—not your personality or something inside you, but about your body—and write it in the space provided.

That wasn't as easy, was it?

We need to develop an attitude of gratitude about our bodies. We need to be able to identify things we love about our bodies and celebrate them in Christ.

> Do you not know that your body is a temple of the Holy Spirit, who is in you, whom you have received from God? You are not your own; you were bought at a price. Therefore *honor* God with your body (1 Corinthians 6:19-20, emphasis added).

God paid a very dear price for you; He gave the life of His only Son, Jesus. Honoring God with your body should be a natural response out of gratitude and obedience. One way we can honor God with our bodies is to have a continuing attitude of celebration and thankfulness for the way He designed us.

CHOOSING AN ACCOUNTABILITY PARTNER

Two are better than one, because they have a good return
for their work: If one falls down, his friend can help him up.
But pity the man who falls and has no one to help him up!
Ecclesiastes 4:9-10

Let's face it—losing weight can be really hard work, especially if you try to do it alone. For many of us on our wellness journey, an accountability or prayer partner can be essential. Just knowing you have someone alongside you can be a comfort. This person may be in your First Place class, but not necessarily. You may choose the equally valuable support of a spouse, friend or coworker.

FINDING AN ACCOUNTABILITY PARTNER

The following Accountability Partner Evaluation will be helpful in choosing a good accountability partner. Before you ask a particular person to be your partner, answer the following questions about him or her. Be as honest as possible. Circle your answers and total your score. Refer to the scale at the end of the evaluation to determine your results.

Accountability Partner Evaluation

1. This person has never had a weight problem in the past but is someone I would like to look like.

    Yes (1)   No (3)

2. Talking about weight loss is a natural part of our conversation and comes easily.

    Yes (5)   No (1)

3. This person would be willing to listen to me, even if I were not experiencing success at weight loss.

    Yes (5)   No (1)

4. This person offers excuses for me when I am not losing weight.

Yes (1)   No (5)

5. This person is willing to spend time in prayer for me when I need it.

Yes (4)   No (1)

6. As I achieve a certain level of success in my weight loss, there is a chance this person would become jealous.

Yes (1)   No (3)

7. This person has the time to invest in encouraging me to keep my commitments to First Place and genuinely cares about my health and well-being.

Yes (6)   No (1)

25-31 Points—You and your potential partner are comfortable with each other and can be an honest encouragement to each other.

16-24 Points—You may have a potential partner, but there are some concerns you will need to address with him or her before you begin an accountability relationship.

7-15 Points—This potential partner is a high risk for you. You will likely be disappointed in the lack of accountability this person has to offer. Keep looking—there is just the right person out there for you!

WHAT DOES MY PARTNER NEED TO KNOW?

Communication is an essential part of any healthy relationship. If you can communicate effectively, you are on the way to a successful relationship. It is important that your accountability partner clearly understands what role he or she is to play in your wellness journey. Here are some specific ideas for making it work:

🍎 **Be specific** about ways your partner can help. Do not expect your partner to read your mind. If you need praise when you do well, but not when you don't, tell him or her. The more specific you are with your request, the better your partner will be able to help and encourage you. "Walk with me three mornings a week" is a much better request than "Encourage me to exercise."

🍎 **Be honest** with your partner. Share your areas of weakness as well as your strengths and make sure you choose a partner who does not have the same ones. For example, if you struggle to make good food choices, choose someone who is disciplined in that area but who may need your encouragement to exercise.

◉ **Be an encouragement** to your partner. A one-way relationship is never successful. Taking time to thank your partner for his or her friendship and time goes a long way in blessing your partner for his or her investment.

Ultimately, we are accountable to God and are responsible for the choices we make. We are told in Hebrews 12:1, "Throw off everything that hinders and the sin that so easily entangles, and let us run with perseverance the race marked out for us." We must run our own race to wellness, but an accountability partner can be the source of the support and encouragement we need to make it to the finish line.

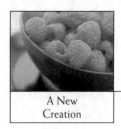

A New
Creation

FIRST PLACE
MENU PLANS

Each plan is based on approximately 1,400 calories.

Breakfast	0-1 meats, 1-2 breads, 1 fruit, 0-1 milk, 0-½ fat
Lunch	1-2 meats, 2 breads, 1 vegetable, 1 fruit, 1 fat
Dinner	2-3 meats, 2 breads, 2 vegetables, 1 fat
Snacks	1-2 breads, 1 fruit, 1 milk, ½-1 fat (or any remaining exchanges)
Daily Total	4-5 meats, 6-7 breads, 3-4 vegetables, 3-4 fruits, 2-3 milks, 3-4 fats

Note: You may always choose the high range for vegetables and fruits, but limit high range to only one category in meats, breads, milks or fats.

For more calories, add the following to the 1,400-calorie plan:

1,600 calories	2 breads, 1 fat
1,800 calories	2 meats, 3 breads, 1 vegetable, 1 fat
2,000 calories	2 meats, 4 breads, 1 vegetable, 3 fats
2,200 calories	2 meats, 5 breads, 1 vegetable, 1 fruit, 5 fats
2,400 calories	2 meats, 6 breads, 2 vegetables, 1 fruit, 6 fats

The exchanges for these meals were calculated using the MasterCook software. It uses a database of over 6,000 food items prepared using United States Department of Agriculture (USDA) publications and information from food manufacturers. As with any nutritional program, MasterCook calculates the nutritional values of the recipes based on ingredients. Nutrition may vary due to how the food is prepared, where the food comes from, soil content, season, ripeners, processing and methods of preparation. For these reasons, please use the recipes and menu plans as approximate guides. As always, consult your physician and/or a registered dietitian before starting a diet program.

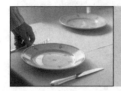

Note: We've included bonus recipes in this study's menu plans. Recipes for *italicized* items in menus can be found in each mealtime section.

☕ Breakfast

1 small apple, diced, mixed with
¼ c. low-fat cottage cheese and
2 tsp. dry-roasted sunflower kernels, served in
½ whole-wheat pocket pita

Exchanges: 1 meat, 1 bread, 1 fruit, ½ fat

~~~~~~

1 serving *Rutti-Tutti-Fruitti Smoothie*
4 reduced-fat Triscuits, topped with
1 oz. sliced 2% sharp cheddar cheese

Exchanges: 1 meat, ½ bread, 2 fruits, 1 milk, ½ fat

~~~~~~

1 c. high-fiber cereal flakes
¾ c. nonfat milk
½ c. blueberries or ½ banana
1 tsp. dry-roasted sunflower kernels or walnuts

Exchanges: 2 breads, ½ fruit, ¾ milk, ½ fat

~~~~~~

½ c. oatmeal
1 c. skim milk
1 dash cinnamon
2 tbsp. raisins
1 tsp. chopped walnuts
  Salt to taste

Combine all of the ingredients in a medium saucepan and cook over medium heat until thickened.

Exchanges: 2 breads, 1 fruit, 1 milk, ½ fat

~~~~~~

½ medium banana, sliced

1 c. nonfat milk

½ c. plain nonfat yogurt

½ c. high-fiber cereal flakes

1 tsp. vanilla extract

1 packet Splenda sugar substitute

½ c. ice

1 dash cinnamon

Combine all ingredients in a blender and puree until smooth.

Exchanges: 1 bread, 1 fruit, 1 ½ milks

~~~~~~

1 slice whole wheat bread, toasted and topped with

1 tbsp. peanut butter and

1 small apple, sliced

Exchanges: ½ meat, 1 bread, 1 fruit, 1 fat

~~~~~~

½ c. blueberries, layered with

½ c. sliced strawberries,

1 c. plain nonfat yogurt and

½ c. high fiber cereal flakes, and topped with

1 tsp. chopped walnuts

Exchanges: 1 bread, 1 fruit, 1 ½ milks, ½ fat

~~~~~~

1 serving *Fruited Couscous*

1 c. nonfat milk

Exchanges: 1 bread, 1 fruit, 1 milk

~~~~~~

1 serving *Granola*

1 c. nonfat milk

Exchanges: 1 ½ breads, 1 fruit, 1 milk, ½ fat

~~~~~~

1 serving *Whole-Wheat French Toast*

1 serving *Orange Slices*

Exchanges: ½ meat, 2 breads, ½ fruit, 1 fat

~~~~~~

1 hard-cooked egg, peeled and sliced and served on

1 toasted whole-wheat English muffin

mustard and low-fat mayonnaise (optional)

½ medium banana

Exchanges: 1 meat, 2 breads, 1 fruit, ½ fat

~~~~~~

1 6-in. whole-wheat flour tortilla, spread with

1 tbsp. low-fat cream cheese and

1 tsp. strawberry all-fruit spread, and topped with

½ medium banana, sliced

1 c. nonfat milk

Exchanges: 1 bread, ½ fruit, 1 milk, ½ fat

~~~~~~

2 low-fat Eggo frozen waffles, heated

1 tsp. reduced-calorie soft margarine

1 tbsp. sugar-free syrup

1 c. sliced strawberries, tossed with

1 packet Splenda sugar substitute

1 c. nonfat milk

Exchanges: 2 breads, 1 fruit, 1 milk, ½ fat

~~~~~~

1 McDonald's Egg McMuffin

1 8-oz. carton low-fat milk

1 c. diced cantaloupe

Exchanges: 2 meats, 2 breads, 1 fruit, 1 milk, 1 fat

BONUS BREAKFAST RECIPES

Fruited Couscous

½ c. dry couscous

½ c. water

½ c. unsweetened apple juice

¼ c. golden raisins

¼ c. dried apricots

1 tsp. honey

$\frac{1}{4}$ tsp. ground cinnamon
1   dash nutmeg

In a medium saucepan bring the water and apple juice to a boil. Add the couscous, raisins and apricots. Remove from heat and let stand for 6 minutes, covered. Drain any excess water from the couscous. Add the remaining ingredients and serve. Makes 2 ($\frac{1}{2}$ cup) servings.
Exchanges: 2 breads, 2 fruits

Granola
1   c. rolled oats
1   c. crumbled shredded-wheat cereal
$\frac{1}{2}$ tsp. vanilla extract
2   tbsp. unsalted, dry-roasted sunflower kernels
$1\frac{1}{2}$ tbsp. frozen apple juice concentrate
$\frac{1}{8}$ tsp. salt
$\frac{1}{2}$ c. raisins

Preheat oven to 325° F. Combine all ingredients in a shallow baking pan. Bake for 15 minutes, stirring every 5 minutes. Cool and store in an airtight container for up to 1 week or freeze individual portions in zip-lock bags for longer storage. Makes 4 ($\frac{3}{4}$ cup) servings.
Exchanges: 1$\frac{1}{2}$ breads, 1 fruit, $\frac{1}{2}$ fat

Orange Slices
3   seedless oranges, peeled white pith removed, cut into sections
2   packets Splenda sugar substitute
$\frac{1}{2}$ tsp. vanilla extract

In small bowl, combine all ingredients; toss to coat. Let stand 1 hour to blend flavors.
Exchanges: $\frac{1}{2}$ fruit

Rutti-Tutti-Fruitti Smoothie

½ medium banana
½ c. 100% orange juice
½ c. fresh strawberry halves
½ c. fresh peeled, sliced peaches
1 c. skim milk

Place all ingredients in a blender and puree until smooth. You may use any combination of fresh fruit or 100% fruit juice. Makes 2 (12-ounce) servings.

Exchanges: 2 fruits, ½ milk

Whole-Wheat French Toast

8 slices whole-wheat bread
1 8-oz. carton egg substitute
2 tbsp. nonfat milk
1 tsp. grated orange peel
½ tsp. vanilla extract
⅛ tsp. ground cinnamon
4 tsp. vegetable oil, divided
4 tbsp. Cool Whip Lite
   Butter-flavored nonstick cooking spray

In shallow bowl combine egg substitute, milk, orange peel, vanilla and cinnamon until blended. In large nonstick skillet, heat about 1 teaspoon of oil over medium heat. Dip bread in egg mixture to coat both sides; add to skillet. Cook 3 to 4 minutes on each side, or until browned, turning once. Repeat until all slices have been prepared. Serve hot.

Serve each with *Orange Slices* (adds ½ fruit exchange) and 1 tablespoon Cool Whip Lite. Serves 4.

Exchanges: ½ meat, 2 breads, 1 fat

Teriyaki Beef and Noodle Bowl

⅓ lb. lean ground beef
1 9-oz. package teriyaki-style frozen vegetables
1½ c. water
1 3-oz. package oriental-flavor Ramen noodle soup mix
1 tsp. soy sauce

Brown ground beef in a large skillet over medium-high heat until thoroughly cooked. Drain and rinse off any excess fat. Return to skillet and add the vegetables and water. Bring to a boil. Break noodles into two portions and add both portions to skillet. Stir in half of the seasoning packet and blend in with the beef mixture. Reduce heat to medium and simmer 4 to 5 minutes. Stir in the soy sauce and divide mixture into 2 bowls. Serves 2 (about 1¾ cup each).

Exchanges: 2 meats, 2 breads, 1 vegetable, 1½ fats

~ ~

Deli Style Roll-Ups

2 6-in. whole-wheat flour tortillas
2 oz. deli-style sliced turkey breast, lean ham or lean roast beef
2 tsp. low-fat mayonnaise
1 tsp. brown mustard
½ c. chopped romaine lettuce
6 grape tomatoes, halved

Lay out tortillas. Spread with mayonnaise and mustard. Layer turkey slice, lettuce and tomatoes on tortillas. Roll up and enjoy. Serves 1.

Serve with 1 small Granny Smith apple.

Exchanges: 2 meats, 2 breads, 1 vegetable, 1 fruit, 1 fat

~ ~

Chick-fil-A Meal

1 serving hearty breast of chicken soup
1 serving carrot and raisin salad
1 serving fresh fruit cup

Exchanges: 1 meat, 2 breads, 3 vegetables, 1 fruit, 1 fat

BBQ Beef Sandwich with Apple Slaw

  2 oz. (⅓ c.) *Barbecued Beef* Recipe (see dinner recipes)
  1 6-in. whole-wheat bun, split and toasted
  3 tbsp. shredded 2% Pepper Jack cheese

Spoon meat mixture onto bottom of bun; top with cheese.
  Serve with *Apple Slaw* (adds 1 vegetable, 1 fruit, ½ fat).
Exchanges: 2 meats, 2 breads, ½ fat

~ ~

Tortellini Parmesan with Roasted Peppers

  1 9-oz. pkg. refrigerated cheese-filled tortellini
  1 4-oz. jar roasted sweet red peppers
  ⅓ c. refrigerated light Alfredo sauce
  1 tbsp. prepared pesto sauce or
  3 tbsp. fresh chopped basil
  2 tbsp. grated Parmesan cheese
     Black pepper to taste

Prepare tortellini according to package directions and drain. In a medium
saucepan add remaining ingredients to the drained tortellini and heat for 3
to 4 minutes. Any leftover mixture may be reheated in microwave for 1 to
2 minutes. Serves 4 (about 1½ cups each).
  Serve each with 1 cup carrot sticks.
Exchanges: 1 meat, 1½ breads, 1½ vegetables, 1 fat

~ ~

Greek Meatball Pita

  1 serving *Greek Meatballs* with sauce, heated
  1 whole-wheat pita, split
  1 serving *Marinated Cucumbers*
  1 medium orange
Exchanges: 1½ meats, 2 breads, 1½ vegetables, 1 fruit, 1 fat

Tuscan Chicken and Beans Salad

¾ c. Tuscan Chicken and Beans, cold
1½ c. chopped romaine lettuce
6 grape tomatoes, halved
2 tbsp. low-fat Caesar dressing
4 low-fat saltine crackers, crumbled

Place all ingredients in a medium bowl and toss to combine.
  Serve with 1 small piece of fruit.
Exchanges: 1½ meats, 1½ breads, 1 vegetable, 1 fruit, 1 fat

~ ~

Roast Beef Po-Boy and Apple Slaw

2 oz. thinly sliced lean roast beef
1 tbsp. low-fat mayonnaise
1 tsp. brown mustard
½ tsp. prepared horseradish
1 4-in. slice French bread, toasted
½ c. chopped romaine lettuce
3 grape tomatoes, halved

Combine mayonnaise, mustard and horseradish and spread mixture onto
each side of the bread. Top with roast beef, lettuce and tomatoes.
  Serve with 1 serving of *Apple Slaw* (adds 1 vegetable, 1 fruit, ½ fat).
Exchanges: 2 meats, 2 breads, 1 vegetable, ½ fat

~ ~

Cheesy Ham and Corn Chowder

8 oz. lean ham, diced
1 16-oz. can creamed corn
1½ c. water
3 medium red potatoes, cubed
½ c. chopped onion
1 c. nonfat milk
1 10¾-oz. can Healthy Request cream of mushroom soup

¼ tsp. black pepper

½ c. (2 oz.) shredded 2% cheddar cheese

In a medium saucepan combine water, potatoes and onion. Cook over medium heat until potatoes are tender. Stir in ham, corn, milk, soup and pepper. Lower heat and simmer 12 to 15 minutes. Add cheese, stirring occasionally until melted. Serves 4 (about 1¾ cup each).

Serve each with ½ cup baby carrots with 1 tablespoon low-fat ranch dressing and a serving of *Easy Apple Salad* (adds 1 vegetable, 1 fruit, ½ fat). **Exchanges: 2 meats, 2 breads**

~~~~~~

Lean Cuisine Skillet Meal

½ any Lean Cuisine Skillet Sensation Meal

Exchanges: 1½ meats, 1½ breads, 1½ vegetables

~~~~~~

Tuna Salad

4 oz. can water-packed tuna, drained

½ c. chopped apple

1 tbsp. reduced-calorie mayonnaise

1 tsp. sweet pickle relish

1 tbsp. finely chopped celery

Salt and pepper to taste

8 low-fat saltine crackers

8 grape tomatoes

In a small bowl, combine tuna, apple, mayonnaise, relish, celery, salt and pepper to taste. Serve tuna mixture on crackers and top each with a tomato. Serves 1.

Exchanges: 2 meats, 1 bread, 1 vegetable, ½ fruit, 1 fat

~~~~~~

Shrimp Salad in Melon Cups

⅓ lb. cooked salad shrimp

⅓ c. low-fat sour cream

2 tbsp. finely chopped celery

1 tbsp. finely chopped onion

1 tbsp. brown mustard
1 tsp. lemon juice
   Salt and pepper to taste
8 grape tomatoes, halved
1 small cantaloupe
8 low-fat saltine crackers

In a medium bowl, combine sour cream, celery, onion, mustard, lemon juice and salt and pepper to taste. Stir in shrimp and tomatoes and toss gently. Cut cantaloupe in half crosswise to form 2 large cups. Discard seeds. If needed, slice about ¼ inch from the bottom of melon halves so that they will sit flat. Spoon half of the shrimp mixture into each of the melon halves and serve with saltine crackers. Serves 2.
Exchanges: 2 meats, ½ bread, ½ vegetable, 1 fruit, ½ fat

~~~~~~

Roast Chicken, Romaine and Strawberry Salad

2 oz. cooked chicken breast, chopped
2 c. chopped romaine lettuce
½ c. halved fresh strawberries
3 red-onion slices
1 tsp. dry-roasted sunflower kernels
1 tsp. honey
2 tbsp. low-fat balsamic vinaigrette dressing
¼ c. seasoned croutons

In a medium bowl, combine chicken, lettuce, strawberries, onion and sunflower kernels. In a small bowl, combine honey and vinaigrette dressing and toss with the salad ingredients. Top with croutons. Serves 1.
Exchanges: 2 meats, ½ bread, 1 vegetable, ½ fruit, ½ fat

~~~~~~

Turkey Chili

1 lb. lean ground turkey breast
1 small onion, chopped
2 celery stalks, chopped
1 medium bell pepper, seeded and chopped

3 15-oz. cans no-salt-added kidney beans, drained
3 14.5-oz. cans petit diced tomatoes, with juice
1 c. water
¼ c. cider vinegar
2 tbsp. chili powder
2 tsp. ground cumin
1 tsp. dried basil
32 low-fat saltine crackers
   Nonstick cooking spray

Heat a large stockpot over medium-high heat until hot. Coat with cooking spray. Add ground turkey, onion, celery and bell pepper and cook until browned. Remove from heat and drain. Return the turkey and vegetables to the stockpot. Add kidney beans, diced tomatoes with juice, water, vinegar, chili powder, cumin and dried basil; bring to a boil. Reduce heat and simmer on low 2 hours. Serves 8 (2 cups chili plus 4 saltine crackers each).

Exchanges: 2 meats, 2½ breads, 2 vegetables, ½ fat

BONUS LUNCH RECIPES

Apple Slaw

1 lb. tricolor prepared slaw mix
2 c. diced Granny Smith apples
½ c. chopped green onions
½ c. low-fat sour cream
¼ c. plain fat-free yogurt
1 tbsp. cider vinegar
1 tbsp. brown sugar
   Salt and pepper to taste

Combine all ingredients in a large bowl and toss to mix well. Serves 4 (about 1 cup each).

Exchanges: 1 vegetable, 1 fruit, ½ fat

Easy Apple Salad

    2   c. cored, chopped apples
    ½   c. seedless green grapes
    2   tbsp. raisins
    1   6-oz. artificially sweetened, low-fat vanilla-flavored yogurt

Combine all ingredients in a medium bowl and mix well. Refrigerate 1 hour before serving. Serves 4 (⅔ cup each).
Exchanges: 1 fruit

~ ~

Marinated Cucumbers

    2   medium cucumbers, peeled and thinly sliced
    ½   c. thinly sliced red onion
    ½   c. fat-free balsamic vinaigrette dressing
        Salt and pepper to taste

Combine all ingredients in a bowl and refrigerate overnight. Serves 4 (1 cup each).
Exchanges: 1 vegetable

🍎 **DINNER**

Crock-Pot Chicken

    4   4-oz. boneless, skinless chicken breasts
    1   small cabbage, quartered
    1   lb. package baby carrots
    2   14.5-oz. cans Mexican-style stewed tomatoes
    2   c. cooked brown rice

Place all ingredients in slow cooker. Cover and cook on low 6 to 7 hours. Serves 4 (1 breast and 1½ cups vegetables each).
Exchanges: 3 meats, 1½ breads, 3 vegetables

Italian Chicken and Vegetables Recipe

2   4-oz. boneless, skinless chicken breasts
1   tsp. olive oil
½   c. fat-free Italian salad dressing
¼   c. water
½   tsp. Italian seasoning
2   c. sliced fresh mushrooms
2   Roma or plum tomatoes, diced
1   large carrot, peeled and cut into ¼-in. strips
1   small zucchini, sliced
1½ c. cooked fettuccine (2 oz. uncooked)
¾   c. low-fat Alfredo sauce
2   green onions, sliced
    Nonstick cooking spray

Spray a large skillet with nonstick cooking spray; add oil and heat over medium heat. Add chicken and cook until browned on both sides. Remove and set aside. Add Italian dressing, water and Italian seasoning and heat over medium heat. Add mushrooms and cook about 4 minutes, stirring frequently. Stir in tomatoes, carrot, zucchini and chicken breasts. Reduce heat; cover and simmer until chicken is done, about 10 to 12 minutes. Combine cooked pasta and Alfredo sauce and heat 1 to 2 minutes in the microwave; set aside. Remove chicken and vegetables from skillet; set aside. Cook sauce over high heat about 2 minutes. Sprinkle sauce with green onions and serve over chicken. Serves 2.

Exchanges: 3 meats, 2 breads, 2 vegetables, 1 fat

~ ~

Greek Meatballs

½   lb. lean ground beef
2   tsp. olive oil, divided
1   c. minced onion
1   c. Italian-seasoned bread crumbs
¼   c. chopped fresh parsley
¼   tsp. dried leaf oregano
⅛   tsp. pepper
½   c. water

¼ c. grated carrot

¼ tsp. salt

4 garlic cloves, minced

1 large egg, lightly beaten

2 c. prepared spaghetti sauce (no meat), heated

2 c. cooked orzo pasta, heated

Preheat oven to 425° F. Heat 1 teaspoon oil in a large nonstick skillet over medium-high heat. Add the onion and sauté 3 minutes. Combine the ground beef, bread crumbs, parsley, oregano, pepper, water, carrot, salt, garlic and egg. Shape meat mixture into 20 2-inch meatballs and place on a broiler pan. Bake 20 to 25 minutes or until done. Meanwhile, heat spaghetti sauce and pasta in the microwave 1 to 2 minutes. Top pasta and sauce with meatballs. Serves 4 (5 meatballs, ½ cup spaghetti sauce and ½ cup orzo pasta each).

Tip: Use extra meatballs for *Greek Meatball Pita.*

Exchanges: 1 ½ meats, 2 ½ breads, 2 vegetables, 1 ½ fats

Easy Crock-Pot Spaghetti Sauce

1 lb. lean ground beef

½ c. chopped onion

½ c. chopped bell pepper

½ c. chopped celery

1 clove garlic, minced

1 tsp. Italian seasoning

1 14.5-oz. can petit diced tomatoes

1 6-oz. can tomato paste

1 12-oz. can tomato sauce

1 c. water

1 packet spaghetti sauce seasoning

In a large skillet, brown ground beef, onion, bell pepper, celery and garlic; drain. Place hamburger mixture, Italian seasoning, diced tomatoes, tomato paste, tomato sauce, water and spaghetti sauce seasoning in a slow cooker. Cook on high until sauce comes to a boil; reduce heat to low and simmer 6 hours. Serves 4 (2 cups each).

> **Tip:** Omit the ground beef to use this sauce in *Greek Meatball* recipe. Makes 4 1-cup servings.

Exchanges with meat: 3 meats, 2 vegetables, 1 ½ fats
Exchanges without meat: 2 vegetables

~ ~

Lean Cuisine with Chicken

1 pkg. Lean Cuisine Penne Pasta with Tomato Basil Sauce
3 oz. skinless chicken, sliced

Prepare Lean Cuisine per package directions and top with heated chicken.

Exchanges: 3 meats, 2 ½ breads, 2 vegetables, ½ fat

~ ~

Chicken and Rice Casserole

1 ½ c. cooked and chopped boneless, skinless chicken breast
2 c. cooked brown rice
1 c. shredded low-fat Monterey Jack cheese
1 12-oz. can nonfat evaporated milk
½ c. finely chopped red onion
2 large eggs, lightly beaten
¼ c. finely chopped cilantro
2 tbsp. butter or margarine, melted
1 tbsp. diced jalapeños
Salt and pepper to taste

Preheat oven to 350° F. Lightly grease a 2-quart casserole dish. Combine chicken, rice, cheese, evaporated milk, onion, eggs, cilantro, butter and jalapeños in prepared casserole dish; stir well. Bake 45 to 50 minutes or until knife inserted in center comes out clean. Season with salt and pepper to taste. Cut casserole into 6 portions (about 1 cup each).

Exchanges: 3 meats, 1 bread, ½ milk, 1 fat

Barbecued Beef

1 lb. boneless, lean top-sirloin steak
2 tsp. olive oil
1 medium onion, sliced and separated into rings
⅔ c. barbecue sauce
1 tsp. lemon juice
Nonstick cooking spray

Trim off any excess fat from meat and cut meat into thin, bite-sized strips. Heat a large skillet over medium-high heat and coat with cooking spray. Add oil and heat for 1 minute. Add onion and sauté for 3 minutes or until tender. Add the meat strips, a little at a time, and cook 2 to 3 minutes or until meat is pink. Stir in the barbecue sauce and lemon juice. Continue cooking until heated through. Serves 4 (¾ cup each).

Serve each with 1 small sweet potato and 1 cup steamed snap peas (adds 2 vegetables).
Exchanges: 3 meats, 1 fat

~~~~~~

Burger King Meal

Chicken Garden Salad with Garlic Parmesan Toast and
Fat-free ranch dressing
Exchanges: 3 meats, 1 bread, 2 vegetables, ½ fat

~~~~~~

Crock-Pot Jambalaya

1 lb. turkey kielbasa, fully cooked and chopped
10 oz. cooked salad shrimp, thawed if frozen
1 large onion, chopped
1 medium green bell pepper, chopped
2 medium celery stalks, chopped
3 garlic cloves, finely chopped
1 28-oz. can diced tomatoes, undrained
¼ c. fresh chopped parsley
½ tsp. dried thyme leaves
½ tsp. salt

$\frac{1}{4}$ tsp. pepper

$\frac{1}{4}$ tsp. red-pepper sauce

3 c. cooked rice

Mix kielbasa, onion, bell pepper, celery, garlic, tomatoes, parsley, thyme, salt, pepper and red-pepper sauce in a slow cooker. Cover and cook on low 7 to 8 hours (or on high 3 to 4 hours) or until vegetables are tender. Stir in shrimp. Cover and cook on high 10 minutes, or until shrimp are heated through. Serves 6.

Tip: This dish freezes well if you have leftovers.

Serve each with $\frac{1}{2}$ cup cooked rice.

Exchanges: 3 meats, 1 $\frac{1}{2}$ **breads, 1 vegetable**

~ ~

Tuscan Chicken and Beans

1 lb. chicken tenderloins, cut into chunks

1 tsp. olive oil

$\frac{1}{4}$ tsp. dried rosemary or $\frac{1}{2}$ tsp. fresh rosemary, chopped

$\frac{1}{4}$ tsp. salt

$\frac{1}{4}$ tsp. black pepper

1 19-oz. can cannellini beans, undrained

1 c. reduced-sodium chicken broth

2 tbsp. julienne-cut sun-dried tomatoes

2 tbsp. cornstarch

$\frac{1}{4}$ c. water

1 10-oz. package Green Giant frozen creamed spinach
   Nonstick cooking spray

Preheat a large skillet over medium-high heat for 1 to 2 minutes. Coat with cooking spray and add olive oil. Add the chicken, rosemary, salt and pepper to the pan and cook 2 to 3 minutes, stirring occasionally. Add undrained beans, broth and tomatoes. Stir the cornstarch and the water together and add to the pan, stirring constantly. Heat to a boil; then reduce heat and simmer 5 minutes. Meanwhile, prepare spinach according to pack-

age directions. Serves 4 (1 ½ cups chicken mixture and ¼ spinach).
Exchanges: 3 meats, 1 ½ breads, 1 vegetable, 1 fat

~ ~

Sweet Orange Tilapia Fillets

 4   5-oz. tilapia fillets
 2   navel oranges
 ¼   c. low-fat mayonnaise
 1   tbsp. prepared horseradish
 1   tsp. seasoned salt
 1   tbsp. honey
 2   c. cooked brown rice

Preheat oven to 400° F. Slice the oranges in half and squeeze the juice
into a medium bowl. Add mayonnaise, horseradish, salt and honey and
whisk until blended. Line a baking sheet with foil and place fish fillets on
foil. Top each fillet evenly with orange mixture and bake 12 to 15 minutes
or until fish flakes easily. Serves 4.

Serve each with 1 cup steamed broccoli and ½ cup cooked brown rice.
Exchanges: 3 meats, 1 bread, 2 vegetables, ½ fruit, 1 fat

~ ~

Oven-Fried Chicken

 4   4-oz. boneless, skinless chicken breasts
 ¼   c. buttermilk
 1   c. crushed cornflakes
 1   tsp. seasoned salt
     Nonstick cooking spray

Soak chicken breasts in buttermilk for 45 minutes. Preheat oven to 375° F.
Combine cornflakes and seasoned salt in a bowl. Roll the chicken breast
in the crumb mixture and place in a baking dish coated with cooking
spray. Bake for 50 to 60 minutes or until chicken is no longer pink in center. Serves 4.

Serve each with a small baked potato topped with 1 teaspoon butter
and 1 tablespoon low-fat sour cream, and 1 cup steamed mixed vegetables.
Exchanges: 3 meats, 2 breads, 2 vegetables, 1 fat

Teriyaki-Ginger Chicken Stir-Fry

1   lb. boneless, skinless chicken breasts, cubed
1½ tbsp. olive oil, divided
3   c. oriental-style frozen mixed vegetables, thawed
½ c. prepared teriyaki-ginger stir-fry sauce
2   c. cooked brown rice

Heat ½ tablespoon of the oil in a large skillet over medium-high heat.
Add thawed vegetables and sauté for 2 to 3 minutes. Remove vegetables
and keep warm. Add remaining oil and sauté chicken cubes for 3 to 4 minutes or until chicken is no longer pink. Add teriyaki-ginger sauce; stir to
coat. Add vegetables to mixture and stir until heated and coated with
sauce. Divide mixture and serve over ½ cup rice. Serves 4 (1½ cups
chicken mixture and ½ cup rice).
Exchanges: 3 meats, 1½ breads, 2 vegetables, 1 fat

~ ~

Apricot-and-Jalapeño-Glazed Pork Tenderloin

1   lb. pork tenderloin
1   10-oz. jar apricot all-fruit spread
¼ c. cider vinegar
1   tbsp. finely chopped jalapeño pepper
1   tsp. ground ginger
    Seasoned salt to taste

Preheat grill to medium-high heat. In a small saucepan combine apricot
spread, cider vinegar, jalapeño pepper and ginger; bring to a boil. Salt the
tenderloin with seasoned salt and grill over medium-high heat for 20 to 25
minutes or until just pink in the center, turning frequently and brushing
with the fruit spread during the last 10 minutes of cooking. Bring any
remaining mixture to a boil and serve as a sauce for the pork. Serves 4.

    Serve each with 1 small baked sweet potato with 1 teaspoon butter
and 1 cup steamed sugar snap peas.
Exchanges: 3 meats, 1½ breads, 1 vegetable, ½ fruit, 1 fat

Chocolate Chip Zucchini Cookies

½ c. reduced-calorie butter, softened
½ c. sugar
½ c. Splenda sugar substitute
1 egg
2 c. flour
1 tsp. baking soda
1 tsp. cinnamon
½ tsp. salt
1 medium zucchini, grated (about 1 c.)
1 c. semisweet chocolate chips
   Nonstick cooking spray

Preheat oven to 350° F. Spray cookie sheet with cooking spray and set aside. In large bowl, cream butter, sugar and Splenda until light and fluffy. Add egg, flour, baking soda, cinnamon and salt. Mix well. Add zucchini and chocolate chips. Drop cookie mixture by tablespoonfuls onto cookie sheets. Bake 15 to 20 minutes or until browned. Makes approximately 3 dozen cookies.

Exchanges: 1 ½ breads, 1 fat

~ ~

Apple Crisp

6 c. cored, sliced and peeled tart apples (about 6 medium)
1 tbsp. water
1 ⅛ tsp. almond extract, divided
½ c. oatmeal
2 tbsp. all-purpose flour
1 tbsp. sugar
1 tbsp. plus 1 tsp. Splenda sugar substitute, divided
2 tbsp. chopped almonds
½ tsp. ground cinnamon
3 tbsp. reduced-calorie butter, softened
½ c. plain nonfat yogurt
   Nonstick cooking spray

Heat oven to 375° F. Place apples in a 1½ quart casserole dish that has been sprayed with cooking spray. Mix water and 1 teaspoon almond extract and pour over apples; toss to coat. Mix oatmeal, flour, sugar, 1 tablespoon Splenda, almonds, cinnamon and butter until well mixed and crumbly. Sprinkle crumb topping over the apples. Bake 30 minutes or until top is golden brown and apples are tender. (Small amount of sugar is needed for caramelization.) Meanwhile, mix yogurt, ⅛ teaspoon almond extract and 1 teaspoon Splenda in a small bowl. Serve Apple Crisp warm and top with yogurt mixture. Serves 6 (¾ cup each).

Exchanges: 1 fruit, ½ fat

~ ~

Baked Spiced Bananas with Frozen Yogurt

  3 medium, very ripe bananas, peeled
  4 tsp. brown-sugar substitute
  2 tsp. grated lemon rind
 ⅛ tsp. cinnamon
 ½ tsp. vanilla extract
  3 c. artificially sweetened low-fat frozen yogurt
     Nonstick cooking spray

Preheat oven to 350° F. Cut bananas in half lengthwise and place in a 13x9x2-inch baking dish coated with nonstick cooking spray. In a small bowl, combine brown-sugar substitute, lemon rind and cinnamon. Sprinkle mixture over bananas. Sprinkle bananas with vanilla extract. Bake 15 to 20 minutes or until thoroughly heated. Serve warm over frozen yogurt. Serves 6 (½ banana with ½ cup frozen yogurt each).

Exchanges: ½ bread, 1 fruit, ½ fat

~ ~

Brownies

  6 tbsp. reduced-calorie butter, softened
 ½ c. unsweetened applesauce
  2 eggs, beaten
  1 tsp. vanilla
 ¾ c. all-purpose flour
  1 c. Splenda sugar substitute

½ c. mini chocolate chips

6 tbsp. unsweetened cocoa

1 tsp. baking powder

¼ tsp. salt

¼ c. chopped walnuts

Nonstick cooking spray

Preheat oven to 350° F. Coat an 8-inch square baking dish with nonstick cooking spray; set aside. In a large bowl, beat butter, applesauce, eggs and vanilla until blended. In a separate bowl, combine flour, Splenda, chocolate chips, cocoa, baking powder and salt; add to butter mixture and stir until blended. Spread batter evenly in the baking dish and sprinkle with the walnuts. Bake 18 to 20 minutes or until top springs back when gently touched. Cool completely on wire rack. Serves 16.

Exchanges: 1 bread, 1 fat

~~~~~~

Mini Lime Cheesecakes

12 reduced-calorie vanilla wafers

¾ c. fat-free cottage cheese

8 oz. low-fat cream cheese, softened

¼ c. Splenda sugar substitute

2 tbsp. sugar

2 eggs

1 tbsp. grated lime rind

1 tbsp. fresh lime juice

1 tsp. vanilla extract

¼ c. low-fat vanilla yogurt

2 medium kiwifruit, peeled, halved and sliced

Preheat oven to 350° F. Line 12 muffin tins with paper baking liners. Place one vanilla wafer in the bottom of each liner. Blend the cottage cheese in a blender or food processor until smooth. In a medium bowl, combine the cottage cheese and cream cheese and beat at medium speed with an electric mixer until creamy. Gradually add the Splenda and sugar and mix well. Add the eggs, lime rind, lime juice and vanilla extract. Beat until smooth. Spoon the cheese mixture evenly over the vanilla wafers. Bake 20 minutes or until cheesecakes are almost set (do not overbake). Allow the cheese-cakes to cool completely on a wire rack. Remove from muffin tins and chill thoroughly. Spread the vanilla yogurt evenly over cheesecakes, and top each with kiwifruit slices. Serves 12.

Exchanges: ½ meat, ½ bread, 1 fat

~ ~

Peanut Butter Cookies

1	c. chunky-style peanut butter
¼	c. butter, softened
1	egg, beaten
2	tbsp. honey
½	tsp. vanilla
1	c. Splenda sugar substitute
1½	c. flour
½	tsp. baking soda
½	tsp. salt
	Nonstick cooking spray

Preheat oven to 350° F. In a large bowl, beat peanut butter and butter with an electric mixer until creamy. Add egg, honey and vanilla; beat on high speed approximately 1½ minutes. Add Splenda and beat on medium speed until well blended. In small bowl, combine flour, baking soda and salt. Slowly add flour mixture to peanut butter mixture, beating on low speed until well blended. Spray a nonstick baking sheet with nonstick cooking spray. Roll the dough into balls (about 1 tablespoon of dough each) and drop onto baking sheet about 2 inches apart. Flatten each ball with a fork, pressing a crisscross pattern into each cookie. Bake 7 to 9 minutes or until light brown around the edges. Cool on a wire rack. Makes 24 cookies.

Exchanges: 1 bread, 1 fat

~ ~

Pineapple Dream Pie

8	oz. low-fat cream cheese, softened
¼	c. Splenda sugar substitute
1½	c. Cool Whip Lite, thawed

1   20-oz. can crushed pineapple, packed in juice, well drained
1   reduced-fat graham-cracker piecrust

In a medium bowl, beat cream cheese and Splenda until smooth. Fold in Cool Whip and drained pineapple. Spoon into piecrust and chill 2 hours or overnight. Serves 10.

Exchanges: ½ **meat, 1 bread,** ½ **fruit, 1 fat**

Conversion Chart
Equivalent Imperial and Metric Measurements

Liquid Measures

Fluid Ounces	U.S.	Imperial	Milliliters
	1 teaspoon	1 teaspoon	5
¼	2 teaspoons	1 dessert spoon	7
½	1 tablespoon	1 tablespoon	15
1	2 tablespoons	2 tablespoons	28
2	¼ cup	4 tablespoons	56
4	½ cup or ¼ pint		110
5		¼ pint or 1 gill	140
6	¾ cup		170
8	1 cup or ½ pint		225
9			250 or ¼ liter
10	1¼ cups	½ pint	280
12	1½ cups or ¾ pint		340
15		¾ pint	420
16	2 cups or 1 pint		450
18	2¼ cups		500 or ½ liter
20	2½ cups	1 pint	560
24	3 cups or 1½ pints		675
25		1¼	700
30	3¾ cups	1½ pints	840
32	4 cups		900
36	4½ cups		1,000 or 1 liter
40	5 cups	2 pints or 1 quart	1,120
48	6 cups or 3 pints		1,350
50		2½ pints	1,400

Solid Measures

U.S. and Imperial Measures		Metric Measures	
Ounces	Pounds	Grams	Kilos
1		28	
2		56	
3½		100	
4	¼	112	
5		140	
6		168	
8	½	225	
9		250	¼
12	¾	340	
16	1	450	
18		500	½
20	1¼	560	
24		675	
27		750	¾
32	2	900	
36	2¼	1,000	1
40	2½	1,100	
48	3	1,350	
54		1,500	1½
64	4	1,800	
72	4½	2,000	2
80	5	2,250	2¼
100	6	2,800	2¾

Oven Temperature Equivalents

Fahrenheit	Celsius	Gas Mark	Description
225	110	1/4	Cool
250	130	1/2	
275	140	1	Very Slow
300	150	2	
325	170	3	Slow
350	180	4	Moderate
375	190	5	
400	200	6	Moderately Hot
425	220	7	Fairly Hot
450	230	8	Hot
475	240	9	Very Hot
500	250	10	Extremely Hot

LEADER'S DISCUSSION GUIDE

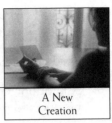

A New Creation

Week One: What Is a New Creation in Christ?

1. **Before the meeting:** Draw two columns on a white board, chalk-board or poster board. Above the columns, write the following headings: "Worldly View" and "Godly View."

2. Read the Nine Commitments and then recite this week's memory verse as a group.

3. Read 2 Corinthians 5:16-17. Discuss what it means to regard others from a worldly point of view. List the group's answers under the column titled "Worldly View."

4. Discuss what it means to have a godly view of others and self. List the group's answers under the column titled "Godly View."

5. Invite members to share how a godly view of themselves can affect their ability to meet their goals and commitments for First Place.

6. Read Ephesians 4:17-24. Discuss questions in Day 3, especially the three instructions we are given concerning our new selves.

7. Close in prayer by inviting three volunteers to pray for God's blessing, God's provision and God's guidance for each group member.

Week Two: Desire to Live as a New Creation

1. Recite the memory verse as a group. Invite members to share what they think delight in the Lord means.

2. Discuss the questions from Day 1. Invite a volunteer to share a recent experience when God rescued him or her from a battle.

3. Have members form small groups to discuss their experiences with praying on their knees from Day 3. Invite members to describe their altar or special place they go to be with God.

4. Bring the whole group back together. Read Ephesians 4:17-19. Discuss ways that our hearts can become hardened.

5. Read Proverbs 4:23. Discuss the questions from Day 5.

6. Ask for prayer requests before closing in prayer. Invite different members to pray for each individual request. Close by giving God thanks and praise.

Week Three: Choose to Live as a New Creation

1. **Before the meeting**: Choose a worship song that you would like your members to hear, preferably one that touches on the themes of this week's lessons. Find a small CD player and have the CD player and CD ready when class begins.

2. As a group, recite this week's memory verse. Invite volunteers to share how their thoughts have been influenced by this verse.

3. Discuss the questions from Day 1. Ask a volunteer to share a time when he or she chose to serve God even though he or she didn't feel like it, explaining how that decision affected his or her heart.

4. Have members form small groups to share their answers to the question in Day 2 regarding foreign gods in our lives. Encourage members to share any struggles they have with getting rid of those idols.

5. Read John 4:23 as a group. Invite members to share ways they worship God.

6. Inform the group that you have prepared a special song to aid them in worshiping God. Ask members to close their eyes and listen as you play the song.

7. Close in prayer by asking volunteers to pray the Scriptures from Day 7.

Week Four: Recognize Your Obstacles

1. **Before the meeting**: On a white board, chalkboard or poster board, write the following headings: "Treasures on Earth" and "Treasures in Heaven."

2. As a group, recite this week's memory verse.

3. Have members form small groups to share their answers from Day 3 about the different thoughts they have regarding their commitments and goals for First Place. Let the members know that they will not be asked to share their answers with the whole group. Instruct the group that as each member shares his or her answers, another member in the small group should say something encouraging to that person.

4. Bring the whole group together. Discuss the questions from Day 4, and then discuss ways that pride can enter into our lives.

5. Invite members to share examples of treasures on Earth and treasures in heaven. List the group's answers under the appropriate headings.

6. Read Matthew 6:33-34. Ask a volunteer to share a short testimony of how this verse applies to his or her life. Be prepared to give your own testimony.

7. Close in prayer by asking each member to thank God for one eternal treasure He has given him or her.

Week Five: Exercise Your Given Authority

1. Recite this week's memory verse as a group.

2. Ask the group to name the four resources God has given us to exercise our given authority, and then discuss how each resource helps us move or overcome the obstacles in our lives.

3. Discuss why prayer is such an important element in reaching First Place goals. Ask two or three volunteers to share how prayer has helped them keep the Nine Commitments this week.

4. Discuss the questions from Day 5. Encourage members to share what God revealed to them concerning what they say about themselves and their lives.

5. Ask a volunteer to share an obstacle he or she is facing. As a group, discuss how prayer, the Holy Spirit, the name of Jesus and God's Word can help the person remove the obstacle or gain strength and peace to walk through the obstacle.

6. Have members form small groups for a closing time of prayer. Have members share their needs with those in their group and then spend time praying for each need. Remind members that they do not need to disclose specific information to the group.

Week Six: Begin the Process of Change

1. **Before the meeting:** Choose several questions from Days 1, 4 and 5 that you think would be especially beneficial for your group to discuss.

2. Recite this week's memory verse as a group. Ask members to share how this memory verse affected their view of approaching God this week.

3. Invite members to share their answers to the questions you selected from Day 1.

4. Read Genesis 3:1-8 aloud. Discuss Satan's methodical plan to destroy Eve.

5. Ask a volunteer to list Satan's tools as identified in Day 2. Ask another volunteer to explain how Satan uses each tool in our lives.

6. Read 2 Corinthians 11:3 as a group and discuss the meaning of this verse.

7. Invite members to share their answers to the questions you selected from Day 4.

8. Read 2 Corinthians 10:5. Discuss how we can apply this verse to our daily lives.

9. Invite members to share their answers to the questions you selected from Day 5.

10. Close in prayer. Invite each member to thank and praise God for one of His specific attributes as he or she prays.

Week Seven: The Heart of God

1. **Before the meeting:** Draw two large hearts on a white board, chalkboard or poster board.

2. Recite this week's memory verse as a group.

3. Discuss the questions from Day 1.

4. Ask members to share how God describes Himself in His Word. Write their answers in the first heart. Then ask members to share characteristics that we sometimes attribute to God but that are not

consistent with His Word. Write their answers in the second heart.

5. Have the members form small groups. Read each characteristic that is not consistent with God's Word, and then ask the members to raise their hands if they struggle with thinking or believing that the attribute is true of God.

6. Have the members pray for one another, asking God to free them from any thoughts or beliefs about God that are not based on God's Word.

7. Discuss any questions that the members have from Days 2 through 5.

8. Ask a volunteer to read Psalm 100, and then close in prayer. Allow time for each member to thank God for what He is doing in his or her life.

Week Eight: Find Healing for Your Heart

1. **Before the meeting:** Ask God to show you a member that He would like to use to share the testimony of His healing to the group. Call the member God lays on your heart and ask the member if he or she would be willing to share a brief testimony of God's healing power in his or her life.

2. Recite this week's memory verse as a group. Ask two volunteers to share how this verse has ministered to their hearts this week.

3. Discuss the questions from Day 2. Encourage members to discuss the assignment they completed at the end of Day 2.

4. Invite the member you selected earlier to share his or her testimony. Have the group pray for this member before he or she shares.

5. Discuss the questions from Day 3 regarding forgiveness.

6. Have the members form small groups. Have one member from each group share a time when he or she experienced freedom through forgiving someone. Ask all the members if there is someone in their lives today whom they need to forgive. They do not need to share the person's name or the offense. Ask the members to pray for one another to receive God's grace and strength to forgive.

7. Ask two or three volunteers to share their experiences with taking a trip to the Cross.

8. Ask members to bow their heads and close their eyes. As you close in prayer, ask members to raise their hands if their hearts are wounded and they need prayer. Without acknowledging the members by name, ask God to heal their hearts.

Week Nine: Break Down Strongholds

1. Recite this week's memory verse as a group.

2. Read 2 Corinthians 10:4-5 as a group. Discuss what strongholds are and why they are detrimental to new creations in Christ.

3. Discuss the questions from Day 2. Encourage members that Christ took all our sins on the cross—past, present and future—and that when we confess our sins, God forgives us.

4. Read James 1:13-15. Ask members to review the lesson from Day 3, identifying the steps the enemy uses to entice us to build strongholds in our lives. List these steps on a white board or a chalkboard.

5. Discuss how we can avoid Satan's work in our lives and keep him from building strongholds in our hearts.

6. Discuss the questions from Day 4 regarding food as a stronghold in our lives.

7. Ask volunteers to identify and share how a stronghold is broken.

8. Pray the Scripture prayer from Day 5 to close. Invite any members who would like to pray this prayer aloud or silently to pray along with you.

Week Ten: Fulfill His Purposes

1. Ask members to recite this week's memory verse to a person seated next to them.

2. Read Philippians 2:1-4 and discuss the meaning of these verses. Ask volunteers to describe what a servant's heart looks like.

3. Discuss questions from Day 2. Ask members to discuss the question, How do we abide in Christ?

4. Have members form small groups to share the various ways they minister to others. If a member is feeling overwhelmed as a result

of ministering to others in his or her life, encourage the other members in the group to pray for that member.

5. As a group, invite members to share what God showed them in Day 4 regarding His blessings. Ask each member to share a blessing that God has given him or her through participating in First Place and studying God's Word.

6. Read Galatians 5:1. Ask members to name things that Christ has the power to set us free from, including anything that Christ has set them free from over the past 10 weeks.

7. Read 1 Peter 5:8-10. Discuss how these verses can help us to stand firm.

8. Close in prayer. Allow extra prayer time for members who would like to thank God for His work in their lives.

PERSONAL WEIGHT RECORD

Week	Weight	+ or -	Goal This Session	Pounds to Goal
1				
2				
3				
4				
5				
6				
7				
8				
9				
10				
11				
12				
13				
Final				

Beginning Measurements

Waist_____ Hips_____ Thighs_____ Chest_____

Ending Measurements

Waist_____ Hips_____ Thighs_____ Chest_____

COMMITMENT RECORDS

How to Fill Out a Commitment Record

The Commitment Record (CR) is an aid for you in keeping track of your accomplishments. Begin a new CR on the morning of the day your class meets. This ensures that your CR is complete before your next meeting. Turn in the CR weekly to your leader.

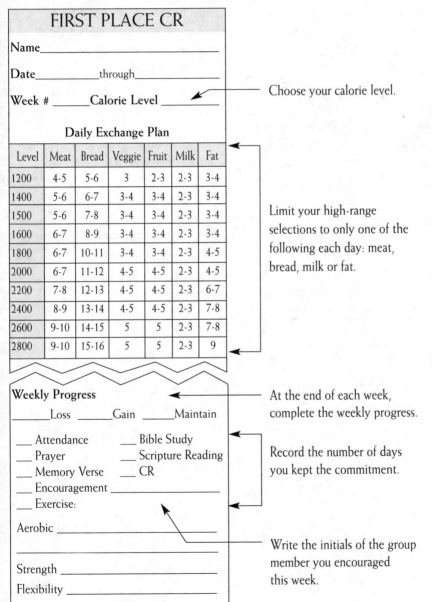

FIRST PLACE CR

Name_____

Date_____through_____

Week # _____Calorie Level _____

Choose your calorie level.

Daily Exchange Plan

Level	Meat	Bread	Veggie	Fruit	Milk	Fat
1200	4-5	5-6	3	2-3	2-3	3-4
1400	5-6	6-7	3-4	3-4	2-3	3-4
1500	5-6	7-8	3-4	3-4	2-3	3-4
1600	6-7	8-9	3-4	3-4	2-3	3-4
1800	6-7	10-11	3-4	3-4	2-3	4-5
2000	6-7	11-12	4-5	4-5	2-3	4-5
2200	7-8	12-13	4-5	4-5	2-3	6-7
2400	8-9	13-14	4-5	4-5	2-3	7-8
2600	9-10	14-15	5	5	2-3	7-8
2800	9-10	15-16	5	5	2-3	9

Limit your high-range selections to only one of the following each day: meat, bread, milk or fat.

Weekly Progress

_____Loss _____Gain _____Maintain

At the end of each week, complete the weekly progress.

___ Attendance   ___ Bible Study
___ Prayer   ___ Scripture Reading
___ Memory Verse   ___ CR
___ Encouragement _____
___ Exercise:

Aerobic _____

_____

Strength _____

Flexibility _____

Record the number of days you kept the commitment.

Write the initials of the group member you encouraged this week.

DAY 7: Date_____

Morning _____
_____
Midday _____
_____
_____
Evening _____
_____
_____
Snacks _____
_____
_____

___ Meat _____   ☐ Prayer
___ Bread _____   ☐ Bible Study
___ Vegetable _____   ☐ Scripture Reading
___ Fruit _____   ☐ Memory Verse
___ Milk _____   ☐ Encouragement
___ Fat _____   ☐ Water_____

Exercise
Aerobic _____
_____
Strength _____
Flexibility _____

List the foods you have eaten. On this condensed CR it is not necessary to exchange each food choice. It will be the responsibility of each member that the tally marks you list below are accurate regarding each food choice. If you are unsure of an exchange, check the Live-It section of your copy of the *Member's Guide*.

List the daily food exchange choices to the left of the food groups.

Use tally marks for the actual food and water consumed.

Check off commitments completed. Use tally marks to record each 8-oz. serving of water.

List type and duration of exercise.

FIRST PLACE CR

Daily Exchange Plan

Level	Meat	Bread	Veggie	Fruit	Milk	Fat
1200	4-5	5-6	3	2-3	2-3	3-4
1400	5-6	6-7	3-4	3-4	2-3	3-4
1500	5-6	7-8	3-4	3-4	2-3	3-4
1600	6-7	8-9	3-4	3-4	2-3	3-4
1800	6-7	10-11	3-4	3-4	2-3	4-5
2000	6-7	11-12	4-5	4-5	2-3	4-5
2200	7-8	12-13	4-5	4-5	2-3	6-7
2400	8-9	13-14	4-5	4-5	2-3	7-8
2600	9-10	14-15	5	5	2-3	7-8
2800	9-10	15-16	5	5	2-3	9

You may always choose the high range of vegetables and fruits. Limit your high range selections to only one of the following: meat, bread, milk or fat.

Weekly Progress

_____ Loss _____ Gain _____ Maintain

_____ Attendance _____ Bible Study
_____ Prayer _____ Scripture Reading
_____ Memory Verse _____ CR
_____ Encouragement:
_____ Exercise
_____ Aerobic

_____ Strength
_____ Flexibility

DAY 7: Date _____

Morning _____

Midday _____

Evening _____

Snacks _____

_____ Meat ☐ Prayer
_____ Bread ☐ Bible Study
_____ Vegetable ☐ Scripture Reading
_____ Fruit ☐ Memory Verse
_____ Milk ☐ Encouragement
_____ Fat _____ Water

Exercise
Aerobic _____

Strength _____
Flexibility _____

DAY 6: Date _____

Morning _____

Midday _____

Evening _____

Snacks _____

_____ Meat ☐ Prayer
_____ Bread ☐ Bible Study
_____ Vegetable ☐ Scripture Reading
_____ Fruit ☐ Memory Verse
_____ Milk ☐ Encouragement
_____ Fat _____ Water

Exercise
Aerobic _____

Strength _____
Flexibility _____

DAY 5: Date _____

Morning _____

Midday _____

Evening _____

Snacks _____

_____ Meat ☐ Prayer
_____ Bread ☐ Bible Study
_____ Vegetable ☐ Scripture Reading
_____ Fruit ☐ Memory Verse
_____ Milk ☐ Encouragement
_____ Fat _____ Water

Exercise
Aerobic _____

Strength _____
Flexibility _____

DAY 1: Date _____

Morning _____

Midday _____

Evening _____

Snacks _____

___ Meat	☐ Prayer
___ Bread	☐ Bible Study
___ Vegetable	☐ Scripture Reading
___ Fruit	☐ Memory Verse
___ Milk	☐ Encouragement
___ Fat	___ Water ___

Exercise
Aerobic _____
Strength _____
Flexibility _____

DAY 2: Date _____

Morning _____

Midday _____

Evening _____

Snacks _____

___ Meat	☐ Prayer
___ Bread	☐ Bible Study
___ Vegetable	☐ Scripture Reading
___ Fruit	☐ Memory Verse
___ Milk	☐ Encouragement
___ Fat	___ Water ___

Exercise
Aerobic _____
Strength _____
Flexibility _____

DAY 3: Date _____

Morning _____

Midday _____

Evening _____

Snacks _____

___ Meat	☐ Prayer
___ Bread	☐ Bible Study
___ Vegetable	☐ Scripture Reading
___ Fruit	☐ Memory Verse
___ Milk	☐ Encouragement
___ Fat	___ Water ___

Exercise
Aerobic _____
Strength _____
Flexibility _____

DAY 4: Date _____

Morning _____

Midday _____

Evening _____

Snacks _____

___ Meat	☐ Prayer
___ Bread	☐ Bible Study
___ Vegetable	☐ Scripture Reading
___ Fruit	☐ Memory Verse
___ Milk	☐ Encouragement
___ Fat	___ Water ___

Exercise
Aerobic _____
Strength _____
Flexibility _____

Name _____

Date _____ through _____

Week # _____ Calorie Level _____

Daily Exchange Plan

Level	Meat	Bread	Veggie	Fruit	Milk	Fat
1200	4-5	5-6	3	2-3	2-3	3-4
1400	5-6	6-7	3-4	3-4	2-3	3-4
1500	5-6	7-8	3-4	3-4	2-3	3-4
1600	6-7	8-9	3-4	3-4	2-3	3-4
1800	6-7	10-11	3-4	3-4	2-3	4-5
2000	6-7	11-12	4-5	4-5	2-3	4-5
2200	7-8	12-13	4-5	4-5	2-3	6-7
2400	8-9	13-14	4-5	4-5	2-3	7-8
2600	9-10	14-15	5	5	2-3	7-8
2800	9-10	15-16	5	5	2-3	9

You may always choose the high range of vegetables and fruits. Limit your high range selections to only one of the following: meat, bread, milk or fat.

Weekly Progress

___ Loss ___ Gain ___ Maintain

___ Attendance ___ Bible Study

___ Prayer ___ Scripture Reading

___ Memory Verse ___ CR

___ Encouragement:

___ Exercise

Aerobic _____

Strength _____

Flexibility _____

DAY 5: Date _____

Morning _____

Midday _____

Evening _____

Snacks _____

☐ Meat _____
☐ Bread _____
☐ Vegetable _____
☐ Fruit _____
☐ Milk _____
☐ Fat _____

☐ Prayer
☐ Bible Study
☐ Scripture Reading
☐ Memory Verse
☐ Encouragement
☐ Water _____

Exercise

Aerobic _____

Strength _____

Flexibility _____

DAY 6: Date _____

Morning _____

Midday _____

Evening _____

Snacks _____

☐ Meat _____
☐ Bread _____
☐ Vegetable _____
☐ Fruit _____
☐ Milk _____
☐ Fat _____

☐ Prayer
☐ Bible Study
☐ Scripture Reading
☐ Memory Verse
☐ Encouragement
☐ Water _____

Exercise

Aerobic _____

Strength _____

Flexibility _____

DAY 7: Date _____

Morning _____

Midday _____

Evening _____

Snacks _____

☐ Meat _____
☐ Bread _____
☐ Vegetable _____
☐ Fruit _____
☐ Milk _____
☐ Fat _____

☐ Prayer
☐ Bible Study
☐ Scripture Reading
☐ Memory Verse
☐ Encouragement
☐ Water _____

Exercise

Aerobic _____

Strength _____

Flexibility _____

DAY 1: Date _____

Morning _____

Midday _____

Evening _____

Snacks _____

____ Meat ____ ☐ Prayer
____ Bread ____ ☐ Bible Study
____ Vegetable ____ ☐ Scripture Reading
____ Fruit ____ ☐ Memory Verse
____ Milk ____ ☐ Encouragement
____ Fat ____ ____ Water ____

Exercise
Aerobic _____
Strength _____
Flexibility _____

DAY 2: Date _____

Morning _____

Midday _____

Evening _____

Snacks _____

____ Meat ____ ☐ Prayer
____ Bread ____ ☐ Bible Study
____ Vegetable ____ ☐ Scripture Reading
____ Fruit ____ ☐ Memory Verse
____ Milk ____ ☐ Encouragement
____ Fat ____ ____ Water ____

Exercise
Aerobic _____
Strength _____
Flexibility _____

DAY 3: Date _____

Morning _____

Midday _____

Evening _____

Snacks _____

____ Meat ____ ☐ Prayer
____ Bread ____ ☐ Bible Study
____ Vegetable ____ ☐ Scripture Reading
____ Fruit ____ ☐ Memory Verse
____ Milk ____ ☐ Encouragement
____ Fat ____ ____ Water ____

Exercise
Aerobic _____
Strength _____
Flexibility _____

DAY 4: Date _____

Morning _____

Midday _____

Evening _____

Snacks _____

____ Meat ____ ☐ Prayer
____ Bread ____ ☐ Bible Study
____ Vegetable ____ ☐ Scripture Reading
____ Fruit ____ ☐ Memory Verse
____ Milk ____ ☐ Encouragement
____ Fat ____ ____ Water ____

Exercise
Aerobic _____
Strength _____
Flexibility _____

FIRST PLACE CR

DAY 5: Date _____

DAY 6: Date _____

DAY 7: Date _____

Name _____
Date _____ through _____
Week # _____ Calorie Level _____

Daily Exchange Plan

Level	Meat	Bread	Veggie	Fruit	Milk	Fat
1200	4-5	5-6	3	2-3	2-3	3-4
1400	5-6	6-7	3-4	3-4	2-3	3-4
1500	5-6	7-8	3-4	3-4	2-3	3-4
1600	6-7	8-9	3-4	3-4	2-3	3-4
1800	6-7	10-11	3-4	3-4	2-3	4-5
2000	6-7	11-12	4-5	4-5	2-3	4-5
2200	7-8	12-13	4-5	4-5	2-3	6-7
2400	8-9	13-14	4-5	4-5	2-3	7-8
2600	9-10	14-15	5	5	2-3	7-8
2800	9-10	15-16	5	5	2-3	9

You may always choose the high range of vegetables and fruits. Limit your high range selections to only one of the following: meat, bread, milk or fat.

Weekly Progress

_____ Loss _____ Gain _____ Maintain

_____ Attendance _____ Bible Study
_____ Prayer _____ Scripture Reading
_____ Memory Verse _____ CR
_____ Encouragement:
_____ Exercise
_____ Aerobic

_____ Strength
_____ Flexibility

Morning _____

Midday _____

Evening _____

Snacks _____

_____ Meat _____ ☐ Prayer _____
_____ Bread _____ ☐ Bible Study _____
_____ Vegetable _____ ☐ Scripture Reading _____
_____ Fruit _____ ☐ Memory Verse _____
_____ Milk _____ ☐ Encouragement _____
_____ Fat _____ Water _____

Exercise
Aerobic _____

Strength _____
Flexibility _____

Morning _____

Midday _____

Evening _____

Snacks _____

_____ Meat _____ ☐ Prayer _____
_____ Bread _____ ☐ Bible Study _____
_____ Vegetable _____ ☐ Scripture Reading _____
_____ Fruit _____ ☐ Memory Verse _____
_____ Milk _____ ☐ Encouragement _____
_____ Fat _____ Water _____

Exercise
Aerobic _____

Strength _____
Flexibility _____

Morning _____

Midday _____

Evening _____

Snacks _____

_____ Meat _____ ☐ Prayer _____
_____ Bread _____ ☐ Bible Study _____
_____ Vegetable _____ ☐ Scripture Reading _____
_____ Fruit _____ ☐ Memory Verse _____
_____ Milk _____ ☐ Encouragement _____
_____ Fat _____ Water _____

Exercise
Aerobic _____

Strength _____
Flexibility _____

DAY 1: Date _____

Morning _____

Midday _____

Evening _____

Snacks _____

____ Meat ____   ☐ Prayer
____ Bread ____   ☐ Bible Study
____ Vegetable ____   ☐ Scripture Reading
____ Fruit ____   ☐ Memory Verse
____ Milk ____   ☐ Encouragement
____ Fat ____   ☐ Water ____

Exercise
Aerobic _____
Strength _____
Flexibility _____

DAY 2: Date _____

Morning _____

Midday _____

Evening _____

Snacks _____

____ Meat ____   ☐ Prayer
____ Bread ____   ☐ Bible Study
____ Vegetable ____   ☐ Scripture Reading
____ Fruit ____   ☐ Memory Verse
____ Milk ____   ☐ Encouragement
____ Fat ____   ☐ Water ____

Exercise
Aerobic _____
Strength _____
Flexibility _____

DAY 3: Date _____

Morning _____

Midday _____

Evening _____

Snacks _____

____ Meat ____   ☐ Prayer
____ Bread ____   ☐ Bible Study
____ Vegetable ____   ☐ Scripture Reading
____ Fruit ____   ☐ Memory Verse
____ Milk ____   ☐ Encouragement
____ Fat ____   ☐ Water ____

Exercise
Aerobic _____
Strength _____
Flexibility _____

DAY 4: Date _____

Morning _____

Midday _____

Evening _____

Snacks _____

____ Meat ____   ☐ Prayer
____ Bread ____   ☐ Bible Study
____ Vegetable ____   ☐ Scripture Reading
____ Fruit ____   ☐ Memory Verse
____ Milk ____   ☐ Encouragement
____ Fat ____   ☐ Water ____

Exercise
Aerobic _____
Strength _____
Flexibility _____

FIRST PLACE CR

Name _____

Date _____ through _____

Week # _____ Calorie Level _____

Daily Exchange Plan

Level	Meat	Bread	Veggie	Fruit	Milk	Fat
1200	4-5	5-6	3	2-3	2-3	3-4
1400	5-6	6-7	3-4	3-4	2-3	3-4
1500	5-6	7-8	3-4	3-4	2-3	3-4
1600	6-7	8-9	3-4	3-4	2-3	3-4
1800	6-7	10-11	3-4	3-4	2-3	4-5
2000	6-7	11-12	4-5	4-5	2-3	4-5
2200	7-8	12-13	4-5	4-5	2-3	6-7
2400	8-9	13-14	4-5	4-5	2-3	7-8
2600	9-10	14-15	5	5	2-3	7-8
2800	9-10	15-16	5	5	2-3	9

You may always choose the high range of vegetables and fruits. Limit your high range selections to only one of the following: meat, bread, milk or fat.

Weekly Progress

_____ Loss   _____ Gain   _____ Maintain

_____ Attendance   _____ Bible Study
_____ Prayer   _____ Scripture Reading
_____ Memory Verse   _____ CR
_____ Encouragement: _____
_____ Exercise
Aerobic _____

Strength _____
Flexibility _____

DAY 5: Date _____

Morning _____

Midday _____

Evening _____

Snacks _____

_____ Meat   ☐ Prayer
_____ Bread   ☐ Bible Study
_____ Vegetable   ☐ Scripture Reading
_____ Fruit   ☐ Memory Verse
_____ Milk   ☐ Encouragement
_____ Fat   Water _____

Exercise
Aerobic _____

Strength _____
Flexibility _____

DAY 6: Date _____

Morning _____

Midday _____

Evening _____

Snacks _____

_____ Meat   ☐ Prayer
_____ Bread   ☐ Bible Study
_____ Vegetable   ☐ Scripture Reading
_____ Fruit   ☐ Memory Verse
_____ Milk   ☐ Encouragement
_____ Fat   Water _____

Exercise
Aerobic _____

Strength _____
Flexibility _____

DAY 7: Date _____

Morning _____

Midday _____

Evening _____

Snacks _____

_____ Meat   ☐ Prayer
_____ Bread   ☐ Bible Study
_____ Vegetable   ☐ Scripture Reading
_____ Fruit   ☐ Memory Verse
_____ Milk   ☐ Encouragement
_____ Fat   Water _____

Exercise
Aerobic _____

Strength _____
Flexibility _____

DAY 1: Date _____

Morning _____

Midday _____

Evening _____

Snacks _____

____ Meat ____ ☐ Prayer
____ Bread ____ ☐ Bible Study
____ Vegetable ____ ☐ Scripture Reading
____ Fruit ____ ☐ Memory Verse
____ Milk ____ ☐ Encouragement
____ Fat ____ ____ Water

Exercise
Aerobic _____
Strength _____
Flexibility _____

DAY 2: Date _____

Morning _____

Midday _____

Evening _____

Snacks _____

____ Meat ____ ☐ Prayer
____ Bread ____ ☐ Bible Study
____ Vegetable ____ ☐ Scripture Reading
____ Fruit ____ ☐ Memory Verse
____ Milk ____ ☐ Encouragement
____ Fat ____ ____ Water

Exercise
Aerobic _____
Strength _____
Flexibility _____

DAY 3: Date _____

Morning _____

Midday _____

Evening _____

Snacks _____

____ Meat ____ ☐ Prayer
____ Bread ____ ☐ Bible Study
____ Vegetable ____ ☐ Scripture Reading
____ Fruit ____ ☐ Memory Verse
____ Milk ____ ☐ Encouragement
____ Fat ____ ____ Water

Exercise
Aerobic _____
Strength _____
Flexibility _____

DAY 4: Date _____

Morning _____

Midday _____

Evening _____

Snacks _____

____ Meat ____ ☐ Prayer
____ Bread ____ ☐ Bible Study
____ Vegetable ____ ☐ Scripture Reading
____ Fruit ____ ☐ Memory Verse
____ Milk ____ ☐ Encouragement
____ Fat ____ ____ Water

Exercise
Aerobic _____
Strength _____
Flexibility _____

FIRST PLACE CR

Name _____

Date _____ through _____

Week # _____ Calorie Level _____

Daily Exchange Plan

Level	Meat	Bread	Veggie	Fruit	Milk	Fat
1200	4-5	5-6	3	2-3	2-3	3-4
1400	5-6	6-7	3-4	3-4	2-3	3-4
1500	5-6	7-8	3-4	3-4	2-3	3-4
1600	6-7	8-9	3-4	3-4	2-3	3-4
1800	6-7	10-11	3-4	3-4	2-3	4-5
2000	6-7	11-12	4-5	4-5	2-3	4-5
2200	7-8	12-13	4-5	4-5	2-3	6-7
2400	8-9	13-14	4-5	4-5	2-3	7-8
2600	9-10	14-15	5	5	2-3	7-8
2800	9-10	15-16	5	5	2-3	9

You may always choose the high range of vegetables and fruits. Limit your high range selections to only one of the following: meat, bread, milk or fat.

Weekly Progress

_____ Loss _____ Gain _____ Maintain

_____ Attendance _____ Bible Study
_____ Prayer _____ Scripture Reading
_____ Memory Verse _____ CR
_____ Encouragement:
_____ Exercise
Aerobic _____
Strength _____
Flexibility _____

DAY 5: Date _____

Morning _____

Midday _____

Evening _____

Snacks _____

_____ Meat □ Prayer
_____ Bread □ Bible Study
_____ Vegetable □ Scripture Reading
_____ Fruit □ Memory Verse
_____ Milk □ Encouragement
_____ Fat Water _____

Exercise
Aerobic _____

Strength _____
Flexibility _____

DAY 6: Date _____

Morning _____

Midday _____

Evening _____

Snacks _____

_____ Meat □ Prayer
_____ Bread □ Bible Study
_____ Vegetable □ Scripture Reading
_____ Fruit □ Memory Verse
_____ Milk □ Encouragement
_____ Fat Water _____

Exercise
Aerobic _____

Strength _____
Flexibility _____

DAY 7: Date _____

Morning _____

Midday _____

Evening _____

Snacks _____

_____ Meat □ Prayer
_____ Bread □ Bible Study
_____ Vegetable □ Scripture Reading
_____ Fruit □ Memory Verse
_____ Milk □ Encouragement
_____ Fat Water _____

Exercise
Aerobic _____

Strength _____
Flexibility _____

DAY 1: Date _____

Morning _____

Midday _____

Evening _____

Snacks _____

_____ Meat ____   ☐ Prayer
_____ Bread ____   ☐ Bible Study
_____ Vegetable ____   ☐ Scripture Reading
_____ Fruit ____   ☐ Memory Verse
_____ Milk ____   ☐ Encouragement
_____ Fat ____ _____ Water ____

Exercise
Aerobic _____
Strength _____
Flexibility _____

DAY 2: Date _____

Morning _____

Midday _____

Evening _____

Snacks _____

_____ Meat ____   ☐ Prayer
_____ Bread ____   ☐ Bible Study
_____ Vegetable ____   ☐ Scripture Reading
_____ Fruit ____   ☐ Memory Verse
_____ Milk ____   ☐ Encouragement
_____ Fat ____ _____ Water ____

Exercise
Aerobic _____
Strength _____
Flexibility _____

DAY 3: Date _____

Morning _____

Midday _____

Evening _____

Snacks _____

_____ Meat ____   ☐ Prayer
_____ Bread ____   ☐ Bible Study
_____ Vegetable ____   ☐ Scripture Reading
_____ Fruit ____   ☐ Memory Verse
_____ Milk ____   ☐ Encouragement
_____ Fat ____ _____ Water ____

Exercise
Aerobic _____
Strength _____
Flexibility _____

DAY 4: Date _____

Morning _____

Midday _____

Evening _____

Snacks _____

_____ Meat ____   ☐ Prayer
_____ Bread ____   ☐ Bible Study
_____ Vegetable ____   ☐ Scripture Reading
_____ Fruit ____   ☐ Memory Verse
_____ Milk ____   ☐ Encouragement
_____ Fat ____ _____ Water ____

Exercise
Aerobic _____
Strength _____
Flexibility _____

FIRST PLACE CR

Name _____

Date _____ through _____

Week # _____ Calorie Level _____

Daily Exchange Plan

Level	Meat	Bread	Veggie	Fruit	Milk	Fat
1200	4-5	5-6	3	2-3	2-3	3-4
1400	5-6	6-7	3-4	3-4	2-3	3-4
1500	5-6	7-8	3-4	3-4	2-3	3-4
1600	6-7	8-9	3-4	3-4	2-3	3-4
1800	6-7	10-11	3-4	3-4	2-3	4-5
2000	6-7	11-12	4-5	4-5	2-3	4-5
2200	7-8	12-13	4-5	4-5	2-3	6-7
2400	8-9	13-14	4-5	4-5	2-3	7-8
2600	9-10	14-15	5	5	2-3	7-8
2800	9-10	15-16	5	5	2-3	9

You may always choose the high range of vegetables and fruits. Limit your high range selections to only one of the following: meat, bread, milk or fat.

Weekly Progress

____ Loss ____ Gain ____ Maintain

____ Attendance ____ Bible Study
____ Prayer ____ Scripture Reading
____ Memory Verse ____ CR
____ Encouragement:
____ Exercise
Aerobic _____
Strength _____
Flexibility _____

DAY 5: Date _____

Morning _____

Midday _____

Evening _____

Snacks _____

____ Meat _____ ☐ Prayer
____ Bread _____ ☐ Bible Study
____ Vegetable _____ ☐ Scripture Reading
____ Fruit _____ ☐ Memory Verse
____ Milk _____ ☐ Encouragement
____ Fat _____ Water _____

Exercise
Aerobic _____

Strength _____
Flexibility _____

DAY 6: Date _____

Morning _____

Midday _____

Evening _____

Snacks _____

____ Meat _____ ☐ Prayer
____ Bread _____ ☐ Bible Study
____ Vegetable _____ ☐ Scripture Reading
____ Fruit _____ ☐ Memory Verse
____ Milk _____ ☐ Encouragement
____ Fat _____ Water _____

Exercise
Aerobic _____

Strength _____
Flexibility _____

DAY 7: Date _____

Morning _____

Midday _____

Evening _____

Snacks _____

____ Meat _____ ☐ Prayer
____ Bread _____ ☐ Bible Study
____ Vegetable _____ ☐ Scripture Reading
____ Fruit _____ ☐ Memory Verse
____ Milk _____ ☐ Encouragement
____ Fat _____ Water _____

Exercise
Aerobic _____

Strength _____
Flexibility _____

DAY 1: Date _____ **DAY 2:** Date _____ **DAY 3:** Date _____ **DAY 4:** Date _____

Morning _____

Midday _____

Evening _____

Snacks _____

_____ Meat ☐ Prayer
_____ Bread ☐ Bible Study
_____ Vegetable ☐ Scripture Reading
_____ Fruit ☐ Memory Verse
_____ Milk ☐ Encouragement
_____ Fat _____ Water

Exercise
Aerobic _____
Strength _____
Flexibility _____

Morning _____

Midday _____

Evening _____

Snacks _____

_____ Meat ☐ Prayer
_____ Bread ☐ Bible Study
_____ Vegetable ☐ Scripture Reading
_____ Fruit ☐ Memory Verse
_____ Milk ☐ Encouragement
_____ Fat _____ Water

Exercise
Aerobic _____
Strength _____
Flexibility _____

Morning _____

Midday _____

Evening _____

Snacks _____

_____ Meat ☐ Prayer
_____ Bread ☐ Bible Study
_____ Vegetable ☐ Scripture Reading
_____ Fruit ☐ Memory Verse
_____ Milk ☐ Encouragement
_____ Fat _____ Water

Exercise
Aerobic _____
Strength _____
Flexibility _____

Morning _____

Midday _____

Evening _____

Snacks _____

_____ Meat ☐ Prayer
_____ Bread ☐ Bible Study
_____ Vegetable ☐ Scripture Reading
_____ Fruit ☐ Memory Verse
_____ Milk ☐ Encouragement
_____ Fat _____ Water

Exercise
Aerobic _____
Strength _____
Flexibility _____

FIRST PLACE CR

Name _____

Date _____ through _____

Week # _____ Calorie Level _____

Daily Exchange Plan

Level	Meat	Bread	Veggie	Fruit	Milk	Fat
1200	4-5	5-6	3	2-3	2-3	3-4
1400	5-6	6-7	3-4	3-4	2-3	3-4
1500	5-6	7-8	3-4	3-4	2-3	3-4
1600	6-7	8-9	3-4	3-4	2-3	3-4
1800	6-7	10-11	3-4	3-4	2-3	4-5
2000	6-7	11-12	4-5	4-5	2-3	4-5
2200	7-8	12-13	4-5	4-5	2-3	6-7
2400	8-9	13-14	4-5	4-5	2-3	7-8
2600	9-10	14-15	5	5	2-3	7-8
2800	9-10	15-16	5	5	2-3	9

You may always choose the high range of vegetables and fruits. Limit your high range selections to only one of the following: meat, bread, milk or fat.

Weekly Progress

_____ Loss _____ Gain _____ Maintain

_____ Attendance _____ Bible Study
_____ Prayer _____ Scripture Reading
_____ Memory Verse _____ CR
_____ Encouragement:
_____ Exercise
Aerobic _____
Strength _____
Flexibility _____

DAY 5: Date _____

Morning _____

Midday _____

Evening _____

Snacks _____

_____ Meat ☐ Prayer
_____ Bread ☐ Bible Study
_____ Vegetable ☐ Scripture Reading
_____ Fruit ☐ Memory Verse
_____ Milk ☐ Encouragement
_____ Fat Water _____

Exercise
Aerobic _____

Strength _____
Flexibility _____

DAY 6: Date _____

Morning _____

Midday _____

Evening _____

Snacks _____

_____ Meat ☐ Prayer
_____ Bread ☐ Bible Study
_____ Vegetable ☐ Scripture Reading
_____ Fruit ☐ Memory Verse
_____ Milk ☐ Encouragement
_____ Fat Water _____

Exercise
Aerobic _____

Strength _____
Flexibility _____

DAY 7: Date _____

Morning _____

Midday _____

Evening _____

Snacks _____

_____ Meat ☐ Prayer
_____ Bread ☐ Bible Study
_____ Vegetable ☐ Scripture Reading
_____ Fruit ☐ Memory Verse
_____ Milk ☐ Encouragement
_____ Fat Water _____

Exercise
Aerobic _____

Strength _____
Flexibility _____

DAY 1: Date _____

Morning _____

Midday _____

Evening _____

Snacks _____

- Meat ___
- Bread ___
- Vegetable ___
- Fruit ___
- Milk ___
- Fat ___
- Water ___

- ☐ Prayer
- ☐ Bible Study
- ☐ Scripture Reading
- ☐ Memory Verse
- ☐ Encouragement

Exercise
- Aerobic _____
- Strength _____
- Flexibility _____

DAY 2: Date _____

Morning _____

Midday _____

Evening _____

Snacks _____

- Meat ___
- Bread ___
- Vegetable ___
- Fruit ___
- Milk ___
- Fat ___
- Water ___

- ☐ Prayer
- ☐ Bible Study
- ☐ Scripture Reading
- ☐ Memory Verse
- ☐ Encouragement

Exercise
- Aerobic _____
- Strength _____
- Flexibility _____

DAY 3: Date _____

Morning _____

Midday _____

Evening _____

Snacks _____

- Meat ___
- Bread ___
- Vegetable ___
- Fruit ___
- Milk ___
- Fat ___
- Water ___

- ☐ Prayer
- ☐ Bible Study
- ☐ Scripture Reading
- ☐ Memory Verse
- ☐ Encouragement

Exercise
- Aerobic _____
- Strength _____
- Flexibility _____

DAY 4: Date _____

Morning _____

Midday _____

Evening _____

Snacks _____

- Meat ___
- Bread ___
- Vegetable ___
- Fruit ___
- Milk ___
- Fat ___
- Water ___

- ☐ Prayer
- ☐ Bible Study
- ☐ Scripture Reading
- ☐ Memory Verse
- ☐ Encouragement

Exercise
- Aerobic _____
- Strength _____
- Flexibility _____

FIRST PLACE CR

Name _____

Date _____ through _____

Week # _____   Calorie Level _____

Daily Exchange Plan

Level	Meat	Bread	Veggie	Fruit	Milk	Fat
1200	4-5	5-6	3	2-3	2-3	3-4
1400	5-6	6-7	3-4	3-4	2-3	3-4
1500	5-6	7-8	3-4	3-4	2-3	3-4
1600	6-7	8-9	3-4	3-4	2-3	3-4
1800	6-7	10-11	3-4	3-4	2-3	4-5
2000	6-7	11-12	4-5	4-5	2-3	4-5
2200	7-8	12-13	4-5	4-5	2-3	6-7
2400	8-9	13-14	4-5	4-5	2-3	7-8
2600	9-10	14-15	5	5	2-3	7-8
2800	9-10	15-16	5	5	2-3	9

You may always choose the high range of vegetables and fruits. Limit your high range selections to only one of the following: meat, bread, milk or fat.

Weekly Progress

_____ Loss _____ Gain _____ Maintain

_____ Attendance   _____ Bible Study
_____ Prayer   _____ Scripture Reading
_____ Memory Verse   _____ CR
_____ Encouragement:
_____ Exercise
Aerobic _____

Strength _____
Flexibility _____

DAY 5: Date _____

Morning _____

Midday _____

Evening _____

Snacks _____

_____ Meat   ☐ Prayer
_____ Bread   ☐ Bible Study
_____ Vegetable   ☐ Scripture Reading
_____ Fruit   ☐ Memory Verse
_____ Milk   ☐ Encouragement
_____ Fat   Water _____

Exercise
Aerobic _____

Strength _____
Flexibility _____

DAY 6: Date _____

Morning _____

Midday _____

Evening _____

Snacks _____

_____ Meat   ☐ Prayer
_____ Bread   ☐ Bible Study
_____ Vegetable   ☐ Scripture Reading
_____ Fruit   ☐ Memory Verse
_____ Milk   ☐ Encouragement
_____ Fat   Water _____

Exercise
Aerobic _____

Strength _____
Flexibility _____

DAY 7: Date _____

Morning _____

Midday _____

Evening _____

Snacks _____

_____ Meat   ☐ Prayer
_____ Bread   ☐ Bible Study
_____ Vegetable   ☐ Scripture Reading
_____ Fruit   ☐ Memory Verse
_____ Milk   ☐ Encouragement
_____ Fat   Water _____

Exercise
Aerobic _____

Strength _____
Flexibility _____

DAY 1: Date _____

Morning _____

Midday _____

Evening _____

Snacks _____

___ Meat	☐ Prayer
___ Bread	☐ Bible Study
___ Vegetable	☐ Scripture Reading
___ Fruit	☐ Memory Verse
___ Milk	☐ Encouragement
___ Fat	___ Water

Exercise
Aerobic _____
Strength _____
Flexibility _____

DAY 2: Date _____

Morning _____

Midday _____

Evening _____

Snacks _____

___ Meat	☐ Prayer
___ Bread	☐ Bible Study
___ Vegetable	☐ Scripture Reading
___ Fruit	☐ Memory Verse
___ Milk	☐ Encouragement
___ Fat	___ Water

Exercise
Aerobic _____
Strength _____
Flexibility _____

DAY 3: Date _____

Morning _____

Midday _____

Evening _____

Snacks _____

___ Meat	☐ Prayer
___ Bread	☐ Bible Study
___ Vegetable	☐ Scripture Reading
___ Fruit	☐ Memory Verse
___ Milk	☐ Encouragement
___ Fat	___ Water

Exercise
Aerobic _____
Strength _____
Flexibility _____

DAY 4: Date _____

Morning _____

Midday _____

Evening _____

Snacks _____

___ Meat	☐ Prayer
___ Bread	☐ Bible Study
___ Vegetable	☐ Scripture Reading
___ Fruit	☐ Memory Verse
___ Milk	☐ Encouragement
___ Fat	___ Water

Exercise
Aerobic _____
Strength _____
Flexibility _____

FIRST PLACE CR

Name _____

Date _____ **through** _____

Week # _____ **Calorie Level** _____

Daily Exchange Plan

Level	Meat	Bread	Veggie	Fruit	Milk	Fat
1200	4-5	5-6	3	2-3	2-3	3-4
1400	5-6	6-7	3-4	3-4	2-3	3-4
1500	5-6	7-8	3-4	3-4	2-3	3-4
1600	6-7	8-9	3-4	3-4	2-3	3-4
1800	6-7	10-11	3-4	3-4	2-3	4-5
2000	6-7	11-12	4-5	4-5	2-3	4-5
2200	7-8	12-13	4-5	4-5	2-3	6-7
2400	8-9	13-14	4-5	4-5	2-3	7-8
2600	9-10	14-15	5	5	2-3	7-8
2800	9-10	15-16	5	5	2-3	9

You may always choose the high range of vegetables and fruits. Limit your high range selections to only one of the following: meat, bread, milk or fat.

Weekly Progress

_____ Loss _____ Gain _____ Maintain

_____ Attendance _____ Bible Study

_____ Prayer _____ Scripture Reading

_____ Memory Verse _____ CR

_____ Encouragement:

_____ Exercise

Aerobic _____

Strength _____

Flexibility _____

DAY 7: Date _____

Morning _____

Midday _____

Evening _____

Snacks _____

_____ Meat   ☐ Prayer
_____ Bread   ☐ Bible Study
_____ Vegetable   ☐ Scripture Reading
_____ Fruit   ☐ Memory Verse
_____ Milk   ☐ Encouragement
_____ Fat   _____ Water

Exercise
Aerobic _____

Strength _____
Flexibility _____

DAY 6: Date _____

Morning _____

Midday _____

Evening _____

Snacks _____

_____ Meat   ☐ Prayer
_____ Bread   ☐ Bible Study
_____ Vegetable   ☐ Scripture Reading
_____ Fruit   ☐ Memory Verse
_____ Milk   ☐ Encouragement
_____ Fat   _____ Water

Exercise
Aerobic _____

Strength _____
Flexibility _____

DAY 5: Date _____

Morning _____

Midday _____

Evening _____

Snacks _____

_____ Meat   ☐ Prayer
_____ Bread   ☐ Bible Study
_____ Vegetable   ☐ Scripture Reading
_____ Fruit   ☐ Memory Verse
_____ Milk   ☐ Encouragement
_____ Fat   _____ Water

Exercise
Aerobic _____

Strength _____
Flexibility _____

DAY 1: Date _____

Morning _____

Midday _____

Evening _____

Snacks _____

___ Meat	☐ Prayer
___ Bread	☐ Bible Study
___ Vegetable	☐ Scripture Reading
___ Fruit	☐ Memory Verse
___ Milk	☐ Encouragement
___ Fat	___ Water

Exercise

Aerobic _____

Strength _____

Flexibility _____

DAY 2: Date _____

Morning _____

Midday _____

Evening _____

Snacks _____

___ Meat	☐ Prayer
___ Bread	☐ Bible Study
___ Vegetable	☐ Scripture Reading
___ Fruit	☐ Memory Verse
___ Milk	☐ Encouragement
___ Fat	___ Water

Exercise

Aerobic _____

Strength _____

Flexibility _____

DAY 3: Date _____

Morning _____

Midday _____

Evening _____

Snacks _____

___ Meat	☐ Prayer
___ Bread	☐ Bible Study
___ Vegetable	☐ Scripture Reading
___ Fruit	☐ Memory Verse
___ Milk	☐ Encouragement
___ Fat	___ Water

Exercise

Aerobic _____

Strength _____

Flexibility _____

DAY 4: Date _____

Morning _____

Midday _____

Evening _____

Snacks _____

___ Meat	☐ Prayer
___ Bread	☐ Bible Study
___ Vegetable	☐ Scripture Reading
___ Fruit	☐ Memory Verse
___ Milk	☐ Encouragement
___ Fat	___ Water

Exercise

Aerobic _____

Strength _____

Flexibility _____

FIRST PLACE CR

Name _____

Daily Exchange Plan

Level	Meat	Bread	Veggie	Fruit	Milk	Fat
1200	4-5	5-6	3	2-3	2-3	3-4
1400	5-6	6-7	3-4	3-4	2-3	3-4
1500	5-6	7-8	3-4	3-4	2-3	3-4
1600	6-7	8-9	3-4	3-4	2-3	3-4
1800	6-7	10-11	3-4	3-4	2-3	4-5
2000	6-7	11-12	4-5	4-5	2-3	4-5
2200	7-8	12-13	4-5	4-5	2-3	6-7
2400	8-9	13-14	4-5	4-5	2-3	7-8
2600	9-10	14-15	5	5	2-3	7-8
2800	9-10	15-16	5	5	2-3	9

You may always choose the high range of vegetables and fruits. Limit your high range selections to only one of the following: meat, bread, milk or fat.

Weekly Progress

_____ Loss _____ Gain _____ Maintain

_____ Attendance _____ Bible Study
_____ Prayer _____ Scripture Reading
_____ Memory Verse _____ CR
_____ Encouragement:
_____ Exercise
Aerobic _____

Strength _____
Flexibility _____

DAY 5: Date _____

Morning _____

Midday _____

Evening _____

Snacks _____

_____ Meat   ☐ Prayer
_____ Bread   ☐ Bible Study
_____ Vegetable   ☐ Scripture Reading
_____ Fruit   ☐ Memory Verse
_____ Milk   ☐ Encouragement
_____ Fat   ☐ Water
Exercise
Aerobic _____

Strength _____
Flexibility _____

DAY 6: Date _____

Morning _____

Midday _____

Evening _____

Snacks _____

_____ Meat   ☐ Prayer
_____ Bread   ☐ Bible Study
_____ Vegetable   ☐ Scripture Reading
_____ Fruit   ☐ Memory Verse
_____ Milk   ☐ Encouragement
_____ Fat   ☐ Water
Exercise
Aerobic _____

Strength _____
Flexibility _____

DAY 7: Date _____

Morning _____

Midday _____

Evening _____

Snacks _____

_____ Meat   ☐ Prayer
_____ Bread   ☐ Bible Study
_____ Vegetable   ☐ Scripture Reading
_____ Fruit   ☐ Memory Verse
_____ Milk   ☐ Encouragement
_____ Fat   ☐ Water
Exercise
Aerobic _____

Strength _____
Flexibility _____

DAY 1: Date _____   **DAY 2:** Date _____   **DAY 3:** Date _____   **DAY 4:** Date _____

DAY 1

Morning _____

Midday _____

Evening _____

Snacks _____

___ Meat	☐ Prayer
___ Bread	☐ Bible Study
___ Vegetable	☐ Scripture Reading
___ Fruit	☐ Memory Verse
___ Milk	☐ Encouragement
___ Fat	___ Water

Exercise
Aerobic _____
Strength _____
Flexibility _____

DAY 2

Morning _____

Midday _____

Evening _____

Snacks _____

___ Meat	☐ Prayer
___ Bread	☐ Bible Study
___ Vegetable	☐ Scripture Reading
___ Fruit	☐ Memory Verse
___ Milk	☐ Encouragement
___ Fat	___ Water

Exercise
Aerobic _____
Strength _____
Flexibility _____

DAY 3

Morning _____

Midday _____

Evening _____

Snacks _____

___ Meat	☐ Prayer
___ Bread	☐ Bible Study
___ Vegetable	☐ Scripture Reading
___ Fruit	☐ Memory Verse
___ Milk	☐ Encouragement
___ Fat	___ Water

Exercise
Aerobic _____
Strength _____
Flexibility _____

DAY 4

Morning _____

Midday _____

Evening _____

Snacks _____

___ Meat	☐ Prayer
___ Bread	☐ Bible Study
___ Vegetable	☐ Scripture Reading
___ Fruit	☐ Memory Verse
___ Milk	☐ Encouragement
___ Fat	___ Water

Exercise
Aerobic _____
Strength _____
Flexibility _____

FIRST PLACE CR

Name _____

Date _____ through _____

Week # _____ Calorie Level _____

Daily Exchange Plan

Level	Meat	Bread	Veggie	Fruit	Milk	Fat
1200	4-5	5-6	3	2-3	2-3	3-4
1400	5-6	6-7	3-4	3-4	2-3	3-4
1500	5-6	7-8	3-4	3-4	2-3	3-4
1600	6-7	8-9	3-4	3-4	2-3	3-4
1800	6-7	10-11	3-4	3-4	2-3	4-5
2000	6-7	11-12	4-5	4-5	2-3	4-5
2200	7-8	12-13	4-5	4-5	2-3	6-7
2400	8-9	13-14	4-5	4-5	2-3	7-8
2600	9-10	14-15	5	5	2-3	7-8
2800	9-10	15-16	5	5	2-3	9

You may always choose the high range of vegetables and fruits. Limit your high range selections to only one of the following: meat, bread, milk or fat.

Weekly Progress

_____ Loss _____ Gain _____ Maintain

_____ Attendance _____ Bible Study

_____ Prayer _____ Scripture Reading

_____ Memory Verse _____ CR

_____ Encouragement:

_____ Exercise

Aerobic _____

Strength _____

Flexibility _____

DAY 5: Date _____

Morning _____

Midday _____

Evening _____

Snacks _____

☐ Meat _____ ☐ Prayer

☐ Bread _____ ☐ Bible Study

☐ Vegetable _____ ☐ Scripture Reading

☐ Fruit _____ ☐ Memory Verse

☐ Milk _____ ☐ Encouragement

☐ Fat _____ ☐ Water

Exercise

Aerobic _____

Strength _____

Flexibility _____

DAY 6: Date _____

Morning _____

Midday _____

Evening _____

Snacks _____

☐ Meat _____ ☐ Prayer

☐ Bread _____ ☐ Bible Study

☐ Vegetable _____ ☐ Scripture Reading

☐ Fruit _____ ☐ Memory Verse

☐ Milk _____ ☐ Encouragement

☐ Fat _____ ☐ Water

Exercise

Aerobic _____

Strength _____

Flexibility _____

DAY 7: Date _____

Morning _____

Midday _____

Evening _____

Snacks _____

☐ Meat _____ ☐ Prayer

☐ Bread _____ ☐ Bible Study

☐ Vegetable _____ ☐ Scripture Reading

☐ Fruit _____ ☐ Memory Verse

☐ Milk _____ ☐ Encouragement

☐ Fat _____ ☐ Water

Exercise

Aerobic _____

Strength _____

Flexibility _____

DAY 1: Date ___

Morning _____

Midday _____

Evening _____

Snacks _____

___ Meat	☐ Prayer
___ Bread	☐ Bible Study
___ Vegetable	☐ Scripture Reading
___ Fruit	☐ Memory Verse
___ Milk	☐ Encouragement
___ Fat	___ Water

Exercise

Aerobic _____

Strength _____

Flexibility _____

DAY 2: Date ___

Morning _____

Midday _____

Evening _____

Snacks _____

___ Meat	☐ Prayer
___ Bread	☐ Bible Study
___ Vegetable	☐ Scripture Reading
___ Fruit	☐ Memory Verse
___ Milk	☐ Encouragement
___ Fat	___ Water

Exercise

Aerobic _____

Strength _____

Flexibility _____

DAY 3: Date ___

Morning _____

Midday _____

Evening _____

Snacks _____

___ Meat	☐ Prayer
___ Bread	☐ Bible Study
___ Vegetable	☐ Scripture Reading
___ Fruit	☐ Memory Verse
___ Milk	☐ Encouragement
___ Fat	___ Water

Exercise

Aerobic _____

Strength _____

Flexibility _____

DAY 4: Date ___

Morning _____

Midday _____

Evening _____

Snacks _____

___ Meat	☐ Prayer
___ Bread	☐ Bible Study
___ Vegetable	☐ Scripture Reading
___ Fruit	☐ Memory Verse
___ Milk	☐ Encouragement
___ Fat	___ Water

Exercise

Aerobic _____

Strength _____

Flexibility _____

FIRST PLACE CR

Name _____

Date _____ through _____

Week # _____ Calorie Level _____

Daily Exchange Plan

Level	Meat	Bread	Veggie	Fruit	Milk	Fat
1200	4-5	5-6	3	2-3	2-3	3-4
1400	5-6	6-7	3-4	3-4	2-3	3-4
1500	5-6	7-8	3-4	3-4	2-3	3-4
1600	6-7	8-9	3-4	3-4	2-3	3-4
1800	6-7	10-11	3-4	3-4	2-3	4-5
2000	6-7	11-12	4-5	4-5	2-3	4-5
2200	7-8	12-13	4-5	4-5	2-3	6-7
2400	8-9	13-14	4-5	4-5	2-3	7-8
2600	9-10	14-15	5	5	2-3	7-8
2800	9-10	15-16	5	5	2-3	9

You may always choose the high range of vegetables and fruits. Limit your high range selections to only one of the following: meat, bread, milk or fat.

Weekly Progress

_____ Loss   _____ Gain   _____ Maintain

_____ Attendance   _____ Bible Study
_____ Prayer   _____ Scripture Reading
_____ Memory Verse   _____ CR
_____ Encouragement:
_____ Exercise
Aerobic _____
Strength _____
Flexibility _____

DAY 5: Date _____

Morning _____

Midday _____

Evening _____

Snacks _____

_____ Meat   ☐ Prayer
_____ Bread   ☐ Bible Study
_____ Vegetable   ☐ Scripture Reading
_____ Fruit   ☐ Memory Verse
_____ Milk   ☐ Encouragement
_____ Fat   _____ Water

Exercise
Aerobic _____

Strength _____
Flexibility _____

DAY 6: Date _____

Morning _____

Midday _____

Evening _____

Snacks _____

_____ Meat   ☐ Prayer
_____ Bread   ☐ Bible Study
_____ Vegetable   ☐ Scripture Reading
_____ Fruit   ☐ Memory Verse
_____ Milk   ☐ Encouragement
_____ Fat   _____ Water

Exercise
Aerobic _____

Strength _____
Flexibility _____

DAY 7: Date _____

Morning _____

Midday _____

Evening _____

Snacks _____

_____ Meat   ☐ Prayer
_____ Bread   ☐ Bible Study
_____ Vegetable   ☐ Scripture Reading
_____ Fruit   ☐ Memory Verse
_____ Milk   ☐ Encouragement
_____ Fat   _____ Water

Exercise
Aerobic _____

Strength _____
Flexibility _____

DAY 1: Date _____

Morning _____

Midday _____

Evening _____

Snacks _____

___ Meat	☐ Prayer
___ Bread	☐ Bible Study
___ Vegetable	☐ Scripture Reading
___ Fruit	☐ Memory Verse
___ Milk	☐ Encouragement
___ Fat	___ Water

Exercise
Aerobic _____
Strength _____
Flexibility _____

DAY 2: Date _____

Morning _____

Midday _____

Evening _____

Snacks _____

___ Meat	☐ Prayer
___ Bread	☐ Bible Study
___ Vegetable	☐ Scripture Reading
___ Fruit	☐ Memory Verse
___ Milk	☐ Encouragement
___ Fat	___ Water

Exercise
Aerobic _____
Strength _____
Flexibility _____

DAY 3: Date _____

Morning _____

Midday _____

Evening _____

Snacks _____

___ Meat	☐ Prayer
___ Bread	☐ Bible Study
___ Vegetable	☐ Scripture Reading
___ Fruit	☐ Memory Verse
___ Milk	☐ Encouragement
___ Fat	___ Water

Exercise
Aerobic _____
Strength _____
Flexibility _____

DAY 4: Date _____

Morning _____

Midday _____

Evening _____

Snacks _____

___ Meat	☐ Prayer
___ Bread	☐ Bible Study
___ Vegetable	☐ Scripture Reading
___ Fruit	☐ Memory Verse
___ Milk	☐ Encouragement
___ Fat	___ Water

Exercise
Aerobic _____
Strength _____
Flexibility _____

FIRST PLACE CR

Name _____

Date _____ through _____

Week # _____ Calorie Level _____

Daily Exchange Plan

Level	Meat	Bread	Veggie	Fruit	Milk	Fat
1200	4-5	5-6	3	2-3	2-3	3-4
1400	5-6	6-7	3-4	3-4	2-3	3-4
1500	5-6	7-8	3-4	3-4	2-3	3-4
1600	6-7	8-9	3-4	3-4	2-3	3-4
1800	6-7	10-11	3-4	3-4	2-3	4-5
2000	6-7	11-12	4-5	4-5	2-3	4-5
2200	7-8	12-13	4-5	4-5	2-3	6-7
2400	8-9	13-14	4-5	4-5	2-3	7-8
2600	9-10	14-15	5	5	2-3	7-8
2800	9-10	15-16	5	5	2-3	9

You may always choose the high range of vegetables and fruits. Limit your high range selections to only one of the following: meat, bread, milk or fat.

Weekly Progress

_____ Loss   _____ Gain   _____ Maintain

_____ Attendance   _____ Bible Study
_____ Prayer   _____ Scripture Reading
_____ Memory Verse   _____ CR
_____ Encouragement:
_____ Exercise
Aerobic _____

Strength _____
Flexibility _____

DAY 5: Date _____

Morning _____

Midday _____

Evening _____

Snacks _____

_____ Meat   ☐ Prayer
_____ Bread   ☐ Bible Study
_____ Vegetable   ☐ Scripture Reading
_____ Fruit   ☐ Memory Verse
_____ Milk   ☐ Encouragement
_____ Fat   _____ Water

Exercise
Aerobic _____

Strength _____
Flexibility _____

DAY 6: Date _____

Morning _____

Midday _____

Evening _____

Snacks _____

_____ Meat   ☐ Prayer
_____ Bread   ☐ Bible Study
_____ Vegetable   ☐ Scripture Reading
_____ Fruit   ☐ Memory Verse
_____ Milk   ☐ Encouragement
_____ Fat   _____ Water

Exercise
Aerobic _____

Strength _____
Flexibility _____

DAY 7: Date _____

Morning _____

Midday _____

Evening _____

Snacks _____

_____ Meat   ☐ Prayer
_____ Bread   ☐ Bible Study
_____ Vegetable   ☐ Scripture Reading
_____ Fruit   ☐ Memory Verse
_____ Milk   ☐ Encouragement
_____ Fat   _____ Water

Exercise
Aerobic _____

Strength _____
Flexibility _____

DAY 1: Date _____

Morning _____

Midday _____

Evening _____

Snacks _____

___ Meat ___   ☐ Prayer
___ Bread ___   ☐ Bible Study
___ Vegetable ___   ☐ Scripture Reading
___ Fruit ___   ☐ Memory Verse
___ Milk ___   ☐ Encouragement
___ Fat ___ ___ Water ___

Exercise
Aerobic _____
Strength _____
Flexibility _____

DAY 2: Date _____

Morning _____

Midday _____

Evening _____

Snacks _____

___ Meat ___   ☐ Prayer
___ Bread ___   ☐ Bible Study
___ Vegetable ___   ☐ Scripture Reading
___ Fruit ___   ☐ Memory Verse
___ Milk ___   ☐ Encouragement
___ Fat ___ ___ Water ___

Exercise
Aerobic _____
Strength _____
Flexibility _____

DAY 3: Date _____

Morning _____

Midday _____

Evening _____

Snacks _____

___ Meat ___   ☐ Prayer
___ Bread ___   ☐ Bible Study
___ Vegetable ___   ☐ Scripture Reading
___ Fruit ___   ☐ Memory Verse
___ Milk ___   ☐ Encouragement
___ Fat ___ ___ Water ___

Exercise
Aerobic _____
Strength _____
Flexibility _____

DAY 4: Date _____

Morning _____

Midday _____

Evening _____

Snacks _____

___ Meat ___   ☐ Prayer
___ Bread ___   ☐ Bible Study
___ Vegetable ___   ☐ Scripture Reading
___ Fruit ___   ☐ Memory Verse
___ Milk ___   ☐ Encouragement
___ Fat ___ ___ Water ___

Exercise
Aerobic _____
Strength _____
Flexibility _____

CONTRIBUTORS

Vicki Heath, the writer of the Wellness Worksheets for this study, is a certified fitness instructor for the American Council on Exercise and a part of their writing faculty. Vicki she is an area director for Body & Soul Ministries, a Christian aerobic ministry, and is the wellness coordinator for her church in Charleston, South Carolina, where she has led a successful First Place ministry for 10 years. As well as being a national speaker and writer, she is a pastor's wife and mother of four. Vicki is passionate about Christ and has a desire to help others understand the value of caring for their bodies as temples of the Holy Spirit.

Scott Wilson, C.P.C., C.E.C., A.A.C., the author of the menu plans for this study, is the national food consultant for First Place. Scott is a certified personal chef with the United States Personal Chef Association (USPCA) and is currently serving in the USPCA as chair of the National Advisory Council. He is also a certified executive chef, member of the American Academy of Chefs (AAC) and a member of the American Culinary Federation (ACF). In addition to his role as a personal chef, Scott also serves as an instructor for the Culinary Business Academy of Atlanta, is on the Culinary Advisory Board of the Art Institute of Atlanta and has recently become the Southeast demonstrator chef for AGA Ranges USA. Scott has published three cookbooks and lives in Cumming, Georgia, with his wife, Jennifer, and their daughter, Katie.

CREATE AN ONLINE COMMUNITY
FOR YOUR FIRST PLACE GROUP!

Now your group can get First Place fellowship and encouragement online!

Myfirstplace.org would like to extend you a special invitation to stay on track with a three-month no-risk trial—a great opportunity for you to make a tremendous impact on your **First Place** group with its user-friendly **website features:**

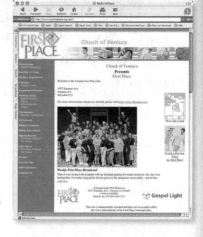

- Home Page
- Customizable Calendar
- Space for Group-Specific Content
- Weekly Devotional
- Bulletin Boards
- Chat
- Publicity Helps

- Online Registration
- E-Postcard Greetings and Invitations
- Group Photo Postings
- Clip Art, Logos and Flyers
- Recruiting Helps
- Group Location Map
- And Much More!

If you'd like to participate in this three-month no-risk trial or to learn more about myfirstplace.org, please visit **www.myfirstplace.org.** After your trial period is over, the myfirstplace.org web tool is just $9.99 a month, or $89.99 for an entire year (a 25% savings).*

*Nonrefundable after 30 days

Register for our FREE e-newsletter at www.firstplace.org

A Must-Have Publication for all First Place Leaders and Members!

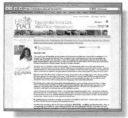

- New Recipes
- Helpful Articles
- Food Tips
- Inspiring Testimonies
- Coming Events
- And Much More!

First Place Group Registration Form

First and Last Name _____
❏ Member ❏ Leader
Address _____

City _____ State _____ Zip _____
Phone Number (____) _____
E-Mail Address _____
Church Name (where group is located) _____
Church Address _____
City _____ State _____ Zip _____
Church Phone Number (____) _____
Church Fax Number (____) _____
Church E-Mail Address _____
Name of Group Leader _____

Three Easy Ways to Register Your Group
Online: www.firstplace.org
Mail: 1957 Eastman Avenue, Ventura CA 93003-8085
Fax: (805) 658-3388

Register your First Place group to receive information about special events and products. **Fill out the form above or sign up at www.firstplace.org.**